LET GO AND LOSE WEIGHT
Releasing Toxic Habits and Beliefs That Are
Weighing You Down

LET GO AND LOSE WEIGHT
Releasing Toxic Habits and Beliefs That Are Weighing You Down

Liz Whalen

The Wisdom Of Wellness

2016

First Printing: 2016

ISBN 978-1-329-87735-1

The Wisdom of Wellness
132 Park Ave
New City, NY 10956

www.TheWisdomOfWellness.com

"Love yourself and all else will follow."

-Liz Whalen

Contents

Preface

As I initially set out to write this book, I began by following the structure outlined for me by my business coach. I created my outline, listed the topics I wanted to cover, and noted some bullets under each to support that topic.

With the outline complete, I wrote the intro, started the first chapter, and then weeks went by and nothing. I always found myself too "busy" to work on the book.

Finally, I sat myself down at my desk, determined to get this book out of my head and onto paper. That's when I realized that it was this organized structure that was holding me back. It stifled my creativity. So I picked up my laptop, moved to a more comfortable spot, and decided to do it my way.

My entire life has been ruled by structure – from growing up with a very strict mother, to joining the military, business school, and then working on Wall Street. Everything revolved around a very structured routine.

Now that I am living my passion and following my dharma, I no longer want or need that type of structure in order to express what's in my heart.

Yes, for certain things, structure may come in handy, but if I am expressing my creative genius, I don't find it very helpful.

I believe that creativity is one of the ways I connect to the divine. It is divine inspiration flowing through me and out into the world. Why would I want to put "structure" around that!

So in order to stop ranting, I will get to my point – sometimes, we need to let go of what we were taught are the rules and start listening to our hearts.

There is an innate wisdom that resides within each of us, and when we learn to tap into that, anything becomes possible.

When we learn to honor our deepest desires, our intuition, and our true selves, that is when we can really make progress.

So I invite you to throw out the rules, throw out all that you've learned, open your ears and your heart and your mind to what I'm about to present to you, and then make the decision for yourself if it feels right.

Feel it in your body – perhaps it's in your gut, perhaps somewhere else. But I want you to sit with the information and then determine how it's resonating for you.

So if you're ready to be blown away by the simple, yet profound truths I'm about to share with you, keep reading. And when you're done, please email me to let me know what you thought and where you feel like you could use more help.

And with that, I present this book to you as an offering from my heart to yours.

To your success,
Liz

Liz Whalen, Holistic Weight Loss Specialist
liz@thewisdomofwellness.com
www.TheWisdomOfWellness.com

Introduction

What Should I Eat?

Most of the time, when clients come to me wanting to lose weight, they ask me what they should eat.

Unfortunately, telling them exactly what they should be eating is not the answer. Because it's not that simple.

If it were a matter of defining exactly which foods, in which quantities, taken at which times were the answer, then weight gain would be much less of an issue than it is today.

But it's more than that. It's understanding what keeps us from sticking to a healthy regimen – even when we know what to do. It's understanding why we crave food as a way to satisfy our emotions (which I will talk more about later), and it's understanding what is missing that we need to address in order to achieve our ideal weight and keep it there.

Excess weight is not a sign that we have no willpower to stick to a diet. It's not a sign that we don't like going to the gym. It's the expression of an internal dilemma that choses to manifest in this way.

Please don't take these as harsh words – everyone, and I meant everyone, experiences internal dilemma. Just some are not prone to weight gain and therefore they don't experience it in this way. But they experience it in their own way.

So the next time you look at a "skinny" person and envy them, please don't. Because you don't know in what way they are suffering. There is no one to envy, except your true self.

Knowing Thy Self

For years I struggled with low self-esteem. I was always self-conscious about my body, about my looks, about my personality. I was completely uncomfortable in my skin. I tried diet after diet, striving to obtain a waif-like figure. I even considered getting plastic surgery on my face because I was so unhappy with myself.

1

"Maybe if my nose was smaller, people would like me better." I would think to myself. "Or perhaps an eye lift to make my eyes appear bigger, that would surely make me more attractive to others."

As I look back on these moments, my heart goes out to the girl that I was. How unhappy she was with herself, and for no good reason.

It's interesting how I can look back on the moments now, completely removed from the situation, and looking upon it as an observer. Completely objective, yet fully empathetic.

These days, I am so full of confidence, I border on the line of narcissism! (Just kidding.....well, maybe ;-)

Since then my posture has changed – I stand up tall and proud; I make eye contact, which I never, ever, ever used to do before; and I manifest exactly what I want in my life, instead of being the victim of my circumstances.

I have a young intern to thank for this. It goes back to my days working on Wall Street – it was during the summer and I was mentoring a college student that came to work for the summer. I'd mentored several before, and was known to be very 'tough'. I wanted them to be the best. To do the best work, to get things right, and to do it all faster than the speed of light!

I put a lot of pressure on those interns, as well as the people on my team whom I supervised. I was a perfectionist and I wanted everyone else to be as well.

This particular intern was pretty cool however. We developed a friendship, while still maintaining the professionalism needed to get the job done. One day he asked me "Why do you always walk with your head down?"

WOW.

I was speechless. I thought about it for a moment, then I replied "I didn't even realize I did that."

That moment changed my life. I realized to myself 'I'm smart, I'm driven, and I can accomplish so much more than I had realized up until that point.'

So I made a declaration to myself that I would never walk with my head down again. And WOW, did my life change!

People started paying more attention to me; they began listening to what I had to say. I was no longer the push-over that had great ideas and a lot to contribute, but never spoke up.

You see, as a child, I was very isolated. Coming from an abusive home, I was never allowed to have any friends over, and never allowed to go to friend's houses. I locked myself in my room to avoid getting yelled at or beaten, and so I became very shy and withdrawn.

This upbringing manifested in several ways for me as an adult, which I'll get more into later, but for our purposes now, this sense of reclusion and low self-esteem was one of them – and it was affecting my entire life!

I didn't have any friends, because I didn't know how to relate to people. I didn't even know what it was like to have friends. I didn't date because I had no confidence, and I isolated myself at work by being the "tough bitch", focusing solely on getting the job done and not noticing that the people around me were, well, people. Everyone was sort of like a machine to me.

Some of them annoying machines, some of them slow machines, etc. And I myself was a machine. I was completely removed from my emotions, and as a result, disconnected from others.

Looking back on it I understand that it was a defense mechanism at play. Of course I removed myself from my emotions, it was the only way I could survived the abuse I'd endured!

My point here is that when life gets tough, we often respond by becoming disconnected. Disconnected from ourselves, and from the people and environment around us.

And this is what we need to address if we are to be successful at reaching and maintaining our ideal weight.

The Inner Game Vs. The Outer Game

Too often, programs focus solely on what I call the "Outer Game" when it comes to weight loss. And not even the entire outer game, only diet and exercise.

Areas that I classify as the "Outer Game" include:

- Nutrition

- Physical Activity

- Digestion

- Sleep and Rest

- Elimination

Based on this list, it's pretty clear that most programs only address $1/6^{th}$ – $1/3^{rd}$ of the total outer game. However, in addition to addressing the entire outer game, it's essential that we start with the "Inner Game" if we want to achieve lasting results.

The areas that I classify as the "Inner Game" include:

- Mindset

- Stress Management

- Intuition

These are the areas ruled by our emotional body, our mental body, and our spiritual body. While it may not seem as intuitive to address these when trying to achieve something that we experience on the physical level, such as losing weight, they are essential because all the different layers of our being are connected, and in order to bring true balance, we must address them all.

If we simply addressed one or more areas of the physical, such as diet and exercise, we'd be missing out on the drivers behind *why* we feel compelled to eat certain things; *why* we have certain hormones in our system that make it harder for us to lose weight; and *why* it's often so hard for us to achieve the results that we're looking for.

The common approach is to think we have a disadvantage in some way, and then to react by catering to the imbalance by treating the symptoms. An underactive thyroid is one example. Instead of understanding the root cause of the issue, and resolving it, we use it as a crutch, or an excuse as to why we can't lose weight.

Once we begin to address ourselves as whole beings, rather than segmenting ourselves (which is the way we are so often brought up in our culture), things begin to fall into place and reaching our goals is no longer a struggle.

So as we begin our journey, it's important to answer the following questions:

- Who are you?

- What do you want to achieve?

- When is your deadline for achieving this?

- Why do you want to achieve this goal?

- How will you do it?

You may find it strange that I'm requesting that you ask yourself who you are, but it's not strange at all. So often we identify ourselves with things we *do*, rather than connect to who we really are.

For instance, you may identify with your occupation, your family role (ie, mother, wife, etc.), a creative passion (ie, painter, writier, etc.); but this is not really *who* you are.

If you lose sight of who you really are, lose the connection with your true Self, this is when imbalance starts to set it; a key factor in weight gain.

In this book, we are going to talk a lot about discovering who we really are. I'll share different techniques that you can use to do this, and we'll explore it from different angles.

It's important that we start with a strong foundation. By skipping directly to the "How" without answering the preceding questions first, success is less likely, because the "How" will be largely determined by the other factors we're about to explore.

So please be patient – if you were expecting me to tell you exactly what you should eat in order to lose weight, please understand that this is a journey, not a quick fix. And that the answers are unique to you as an individual.

What I'm going to present instead, is a road map for you to plot your own journey, the one that is the best path for you. The one that will bring you results without struggle or frustration, and that will last a lifetime.

Let Go and Lose Weight

So with that, let's dive in.

PART I: THE TOXIC BELIEFS

Chapter One | Toxic Belief # 1: Losing Weight is Hard

More often than not, it may feel like losing weight and keeping it off is a constant struggle. Well, I'm delighted to tell you that it doesn't have to be! Once you know what's driving it and what to do about it, it all becomes relatively simple.

I can say this from experience. For years I struggled to manage my weight; constantly dieting, trying new exercise programs, and never really finding balance. I often felt deprived, miserable, and just plain frustrated. Why was keeping the weight off so hard!?

Most of the men and women I coach have had the same type of experience. They've tried diet after diet, only to lose weight temporarily and then gain in back. There has to be a more permanent solution that doesn't feel like torture!

Luckily, through my practice and studies in yoga, Ayurveda, and brain science, I've found a lasting way to reach and achieve my ideal weight, without struggle or deprivation, and I'm delighted to be able to share it with the men and women I coach in my private practice and group programs.

I call it *"Let Go and Lose Weight"*, which is the title of this book as well. As you go through these chapters, you'll come to understand why I gave it this name. It has many deeper meanings, but I'll let you decide which resonates most for you. And at the end, I'll give you some information on how you can work with me further if you're interested.

But my hormones are out of wack / I have a thyroid disorder

This is one of the common complaints I hear in my practice. And with good reason – our modern lifestyles can definitely throw our hormones out of balance!

Hypothyroidism, a common disorder in which the thyroid does not produce enough thyroid hormone, is often blamed with weight gain, as the thyroid hormone regulates various functions, including the rate at which the body metabolizes food.

From an Ayurvedic perspective, hypothyroidism is a disorder in *meda dhatu* (the tissue layer that regulates fat and hormones). An imbalanced lifestyle can cause certain disorders to arise. Some of the common culprits that drive this type of imbalance include:

- Eating too much fat or sugar

- Eating late at night

- Eating foods that are heavy and hard to digest such as meat and cheese

- Impure oils such as non-organic and refined oils; vegetable oils; genetically modified canola oil

- Drugs and medications that disturb sugar metabolism

- Pesticides and other fat-soluble chemical toxins

Of course, there may be other causes that are beyond our control, but the partial list above gives us some insight as to the lifestyle choices that can lead to or aggravate this condition.

Now, instead of feeling hopeless and doomed to a life of being overweight, what if I told you that you could make changes to help bring your hormones back into balance? How would that make you feel?

Good I hope! Excited, inspired – any of these will do ☺

Here is a list of a few things you can do to start bringing *meda dhatu* back into balance:

- Regular exercise

- Avoiding sugar and white flour

- Eating organic

- Eating healthy oils – those which are organic including unrefined olive oil and ghee

- Eating lots of green, leafy vegetables

Now, some of the things on this list, such as exercise and eating green veggies may not seem immediately appealing, but that is what I'm going to help you with as we go through this book.

There have been times in my past where I enjoyed working out, and other times where I absolutely dreaded it and didn't have an ounce of energy or motivation to even consider it. Through my experiences, I've learned the factors which can make exercising something that is enjoyable, nourishing, and that makes you feel great and that you look forward to.

I'll get to that in a later chapter, as we certainly don't want to feel depleted from exercise, and we don't want to force ourselves to do something we dread!

I'll also teach you some tips and tricks for cultivating healthier eating habits, including eating more green veggies, that don't leave you feeling like you're eating bland diet food. Food should most certainly be enjoyed, and I'll tell more about how to enjoy healthy, delicious food that nourishes on all levels in chapter 3.

I have so many exciting goodies to share with you in this book, but for now, I would like you to rest assured that losing weight does not need to be hard.

It does not need to be a struggle, and I'm going to show you exactly what to do to make sure that it isn't. Once you begin to release the toxic habits and beliefs I take you through in this book, you'll begin to see the weight falling off almost effortlessly, and will look at weight management in a whole new light.

I remember when I was in the military, I was so young, only 17 when I joined, and right before I went in, I gained over 15 lbs! Instead of the freshman fifteen, I gained the Marine Corps fifteen :s

Looking back on the situation, I see that it was due to stress. I was so scared to go off to bootcamp, and I became very imbalanced as a result. Once I got there, the stress did not alleviate, but instead it became worse.

During my time in the military, I was always hovering right past my maximum allowed weight. We had periodic weigh-ins, and if I didn't make my weight, I'd have to join a special exercise program that met at 4am every morning! I certainly did not want to have to wake up to exercise at 4am, especially with the long day of work to follow.

So each time I heard that a weigh in was coming up, I'd basically fast for a few days in order to quickly drop just enough weight to meet my limit. I remember how miserable I was each time I had to do this. I was absolutely starving!

But after the weight in, I'd start eating again, and would go right back to the higher weight, which was more than 15 pounds over my normal pre-military weight. I still exercised (occasionally), but I could never seem to get myself back to my normal weight.

When I finally got out of the military a few years later, I instantly dropped about 10 pounds without trying too hard. I just naturally made healthier choices, and was under a lot less stress.

I was amazed at how quickly my body could change just from being in a better state of mind.

Prior to that, I remember times when I was so unhappy in the military that I'd literally stuff my face with every type of junk food I had always loved and found comforting, but still I didn't feel satisfied. I would sometimes eat until I was sick, just striving to quell the feelings of anxiety and depression I was experiencing from being in that environment.

But food was never the answer. As much as I felt it was the only thing I had to look forward to, it never actually made me feel better, and it never satisfied my deeper emotional needs.

I look back on these times when I felt so stuck, so hopeless, and so frustrated, and I'm just so grateful that I've made it to where I am now.

Fast forward to today where weight management is a non-issue for me - it's so amazing, and truly freeing. For the past few years, since I started practicing Ayurveda, I've never had to give my weight a second thought.

I effortlessly maintain my ideal weight, which is actually a couple of pounds less than what I weighed in high school! Cravings and food addiction are a thing of the past for me, and I've seen an improve so many other areas of my health as well.

My skin is healthier, my energy levels are higher, I have a ton of self-confidence, and I don't get any of the symptoms of indigestion that I used to get in the past. As an added bonus, I rarely ever get sick.

I'll tell you more about my journey as we go along, and share the insights I've learned along the way. It is my goal that through this book, you can skip the years of trial and error that it took me to figure this all out, and finally find a safe, effective system for effortless weight management.

So stick around and keep reading; I have so many amazing things to share with you, I can't wait to reveal it all and contribute to the profound transformation you are destined to experience.

On Emotional Eating

Emotional eating is something that an overwhelming majority of people struggle with at some point in their lives. I would say about 90% of the clients I've worked with struggle with it, and I did for most of my life.

As I described earlier, I remember a time when I would eat non-stop just to try to ease my stress, anxiety, and sadness. Then, when I was working in a corporate environment, I found myself eating out of boredom because I was not being mentally or creatively stimulated by the work I did. I found it very dry and unappealing, and so the only thing I felt I had to look forward to in my day were my meals and snacks!

I ate when I wasn't even hungry - either because the hand on the clock indicated that it was time to have a snack, or I'd just grab something to nibble on our of sheer boredom to help me get through the work day.

As a result, my digestion was a mess! I had so much gas and bloating, my stomach was in constant pain. I had no energy, I felt tired all the time. And, I often suffered from constipation. Not a happy combo!

I learned later through my studies in Ayurveda about the havoc stress and constant snacking can wreak on digestion. It all makes so much sense to me now, and I will share more about this in future chapters, but for now I'd like to focus on the impact of emotions on our eating habits.

Please take a moment to think about when you eat due to an emotion vs. true hunger. If you add up all the times you eat and then put them into one of these two categories, which one comes out greater?

Common emotions that can lead us to eat when we're not truly hungry include:

- Stress
- Boredom
- Sadness
- Loneliness
- Worry
- Fear

This is not a comprehensive list, but it should give you an idea of the variety of emotions that play into this.

There are different ways that emotions may trigger us to eat – they may create a "false hunger" in which we think we are truly hungry when we're not; they may cause cravings for unhealthy foods, leading us to make poor food choices, and to eat when we are not hungry just because we are craving something; we may also turn to food because we're seeking pleasure where we're not getting it elsewhere in our lives.

But food is not the answer to satisfying these emotions. In order to end emotional eating, we must address the emotions for what they are, and stop trying to cover them up with food.

Sometimes I see other recommend that you do other activities to distract yourself when the urge to eat out of emotions come up. I invite you to do the opposite. Rather than distracting yourself, I would like you to embrace the pain. Embrace it, look it in the face, and ask it where it's coming from. And then transform it.

I know it might be scary at first, but true transformation often is.

Sharing my story was very scary for me at first, but I knew it would help people. And this has helped me transform not only myself, but the lives of countless others. We never truly know the full impact we make when we follow our hearts.

By being brave and addressing the emotions head-on, we can make profound shifts and transformation in our lives. I wouldn't be here today helping so many people if I was unable to face my emotions years ago.

I'm going to share some techniques that will help you to do this, and also to begin to bring awareness to when you are eating out of emotions. After doing these practices for some time, food will no longer have the power over you that it does now, and you will be free from the chains of emotional eating.

Being With Your Feelings

The first step is to pause for a moment when you're about to eat something and identify whether you want to eat out of true hunger, or as a result of emotions.

If you've determined that its emotionally driven, below is an exercise you can do to work through it:

- Sit up tall, in a chair is fine, making sure that your spine is erect.

You can place a pillow or folded up blanket behind your lower back for support.

- As you sit up nice and tall, let your shoulders gently draw open and back to expand through your collarbone, opening through your heart.

- Think about the crown of your head gently lifting up as your chin draws in and back slightly to lengthen through the back of your neck.

- Tuck your pelvis under just slightly, by drawing your tailbone in and down, lengthening through the lower back.

- Now, become aware of your breath, and feel it begin to become more expansive. The inhalation is fuller and more satisfying, the exhalation is more complete.

- Take a few of these full, deep, satisfying breaths, and as you exhale, feel yourself releasing any tensions, any worries, any cares.

- As you inhale, imagine you are taking in all the healing vibrations from the universe and allowing them to permeate deep into your cells.

- Continue until you feel completely relaxed in your body and mind.

- Once you are fully relaxed, let your breathing return to normal.

- Now I'd like you to ask yourself the question "What am I feeling?"

- Ask yourself mentally, three times "What am I feeling?"

- Allow yourself to feel whatever it is that you're feeling, and then try to experience yourself feeling it.

- So you are to take an objective perspective now and simply become aware that you are a person who is experiencing a feeling. However, you are not that feeling; but rather, it is an experience you are having.

- Sit with this for some time, quietly observing, without judgement. Just becoming more and more aware.

(visit http://www.TheWisdomOfWellness.com/Resources to access the recorded version of this exercise).

What did you discover during this process? Feel free to jot it down in a notebook or journal.

As you set aside time for daily reflection, and start to bring more self-awareness to your feelings and actions, you can make huge strides toward our goals. So I encourage you to make this a daily ritual.

Information Overload

There is so much information available these days, and so much of it conflicts – how is anyone supposed to know what to do!? Is gluten-free the best, paleo, vegan, or whatever else is going on this week??

Rest assured, I'm going to help you clear the confusion. Whew! ☺

The technique I offer is not to follow any specific diet for the sake of its purported benefits, but rather to *learn to listen to what your body is telling you it needs*.

Your body are so intelligent, but through the fast pace of a modern lifestyle, many of us have lost this inherent connection with it. I am going to show you some ways to help you reconnect, and once you do, you'll no longer have to worry about trying to sort through tons of information and figure out which is the right path to choose, as you will simply *know* what your body needs.

And that will likely vary over time. Ayurveda teaches us how to not only listen to our bodies, but how to flow with the environment, which includes the seasons and other external conditions. (It really all comes back to listening to your body, as your body will know what is needed in different circumstances).

Intuition

The first step in being able to listen to your body and decipher what it is telling you is to hone our intuition. Some may think of this as an elusive, abstract idea, however, I see it as one of the basic senses. So often, we are trained to only consider that which we can experience through sight, sound, touch, hearing and taste. If we limit ourselves to these five senses, we are missing out on a hold world of opportunity!

One of the main reasons people tend to gain weight is because they become disconnected from their bodies. We lose the ability to listen to what our body is telling us it needs, whether it be in the form of something physical, emotional, or spiritual.

We stop nourishing ourselves properly, not only in the form of food, but in the form of self-nurturing, intellectual pursuit, creativity, and so forth. We then feel a lack in one or more of these areas, and as a result, we start to crave satisfaction in a way that we know is easy to access – through food.

Unfortunately, food is not usually the answer we are seeking, and so we continue to feel unfulfilled and lacking in some way. And to our dismay, the food we tend to choose at these times is not usually the healthiest and can contribute to weight gain (later in the book I will explain why it's not only the food choices we make that are important, but also the timing, preparation, and other factors including our emotional state when eating that are important).

It can be daunting when trying to remember a specific list of foods that you should or should not eat, which is what many people try to do when they are first introduced to Ayurveda, or when trying to follow any regimented diet for that matter.

However, I'm going to show you a way to tap into your body's intuitive powers to let it guide you to know what you should be eating. We will also explore how you can tap into your intuition to discover what else you might be craving on a deeper, emotional, mental, or spiritual level that once properly address, will end the false hunger and cravings for unhealthy foods.

Silence

The best way to begin to access your intuition is to take some time for silence. Meditation is excellent, but even taking some time out to just enjoy some peace and quiet can be very helpful. It's important that we do this each day.

Most of us have so much going on in our lives, so much activity, responsibility and stimulation, that without some quiet time to reconnect, we can very easily lose that connection with our higher selves and our intuition.

So if you don't currently have a silent practice, I encourage you to pick a time to do so and make it a point to do it every day. You can schedule it into your calendar and give it the priority of any other important appointment. This is the best technique I know for staying consistent with something.

Program it into your phone if need be, or set yourself an alarm so you don't forget.

You might want to choose a time early in the morning before the day begins, or at night before you go to bed. Eventually, you can work up to doing both. Another great time is during the transition from day to night; if you work a 9 – 5, it would be right as you are ending your workday.

By taking the opportunity to process and let go of the activities and experiences from the day, we can move into the evening refreshed and fully present instead of carrying other things with us mentally. (The same concept applies to right before bed as well, we can enter sleep with a clear head and experience more deep, satisfying rest. More on that in another chapter).

Which brings me to my next point – the more we can stay present, the more we can stay connected to ourselves and the world around us.

So often, we live in our head. Regretting or replaying the past, or worrying about the future. When in fact, the only moment that is real is the present moment.

When we take time for silence, it is important that we try to stay as present as possible and experience the moment. At first, you may need to take a few minutes to allow yourself to process all that you've experienced in your day up until that point, but tried not to be carried away into an endless daydream.

If there is something you need to revisit to figure it out or bring closure to, by all means, do so, but don't get caught up with it so that it takes over. Be with it, and then let it go.

Once your mind has settled down a bit, it's nice to bring your attention onto the natural breath. It can serve as a guidepost for your focused awareness. If you prefer, you can light a candle and use the flame to focus on.

From there, just relax your body and allow your attention to return to the breath (or the candle if you're using it) each time it begins to draw away. Don't worry about forcing yourself to stay focused, as the mind will wander, because that's what it does, but rather, become aware each time it starts to wonder, and gently guide it back to the present using the breath (or candle).

Try to do this for a few minutes each day, building up to 20 minutes at a time eventually. But work in increments. Start small and add on.

In addition to staying present during your meditation, it's important to try to be present throughout your day as well.

A good tip if you have a lot to remember that you need to get done, is to write it all down, and check it off as you go. That way you don't have to keep everything in your head, and you can allow yourself to be more present. This is a useful technique if you have trouble falling asleep at night also – jot down all the things that are on your mind in order to release them, then try to clear your mind, knowing you can come back to them tomorrow, but for now it is time to rest. We'll go into this further in a later chapter.

As you begin to bring more presence and awareness into everything you do, you will naturally find yourself connecting with your intuitive abilities. Only when we are present can we listen to what our bodies and the universe are trying to tell us.

For instance, let's say you have an important decision to make, and you're just not sure which way to go with it. You can rationalize it for eternity and try to justify the logic for either decision, or, you can do that briefly, and then allow yourself to feel the different options in your body.

The way to do this is to think of picking one of the options, and then listen to what your body tells you. How does it feel, is there a sensation somewhere in particular? Do you feel discomfort and uneasy? If so, that is probably not the right decision. Do you feel slightly nervous, yet excited and invigorated? If so, this is probably the decision that would best serve you. Your body will tell you if you only listen.

The same technique can be applied to anything, including the foods that we eat. This is why I encourage my clients to try not to get too caught up on lists of foods that are on or off limits. Instead, as you tap into this power of intuition, you can let your body guide you as to what it needs for nourishment – the types of foods, the portions, the preparation, and so forth. It's the best indication for when, how much, and what to eat.

I don't know about you, but that sounds a lot better to me than forcing myself to follow a strict eating plan that someone else assigns for me! And the beauty of it is that we are all unique, and our bodies will require different things for optimum nourishment. This is why a "one size fits all" approach to nutrition and dieting does not work.

And we are not machines. It's not as simple as calories in vs. calories out. There are so many additional factors that go into play, which we will discuss throughout this book. And as we go along, I encourage you to focus on one thing at a time, making small changes, and gradually adding more. If we move too fast and make too many changes at once, our bodies will not like it, and they will rebel against us and our efforts will be shorted lived.

So the best advice is to be gentle with yourself while trying to stay consistent. And if you mess up, so what. We're human, we are not going to do everything perfectly all the time. Just do your best, and come back to your new practices.

The Hunger Meditation

Let's talk a little more about allowing our intuition to guide what and how much we eat. There is a technique I teach to my clients which I call the *Hunger Meditation*. It was introduced to me by my first teacher of Ayurveda, Dr. Bhaswati Bhattacharya.

It is done by pausing before your meals, getting into a comfortable, meditative state as we described above, and then dropping your full awareness down into your stomach.

Once you've made this connection with your stomach, ask it what it wants. Is it truly hungry for food? If so, how hungry on a scale from 1 – 10, with 10 being absolutely ravenous, and 1 being not hungry. Ideally, you'll want to be at around a 7 or 8 before eating. If you allow your hunger to go past this, you've either waited too long to eat, or you have what is known in Ayurveda as *tikshna agni*, and your digestive fire is burning too hot! (If the latter is true, I would recommend working with a practitioner to bring it back into balance).

Once you've determined your hunger level, if you're at a sufficient level of hunger to eat, ask your stomach what it wants to eat. Be specific, considering tastes: sweet, sour, salt, bitter, pungent, and astringent; textures: rough, soft, oily, dry, liquid, firm, etc.; and anything else that may come to mind.

Once you have a good idea of what your body wants to eat, try to choose a meal that fits this description in order to give your body what it needs. Now, this may take a little bit of advance planning if you are not near your kitchen, or perhaps you are dining out and have a variety to choose from. Either way, do your best to practice this exercise each time you eat, and then modify your meal as much as you can within your control to satisfy your body's needs.

Note: Please try to choose the healthy choices if you're having a desire for a particular taste or texture. For instance, if you are craving salt, try not to grab a bag of chips, but rather maybe you have something that is naturally on the saltier side such as seaweed, or you can add some natural sea salt to your meal.

(We'll get more into cravings and what they mean in Chapter 3).

Chapter Two | Toxic Belief # 2: I Hate the Way I look, I'll Never Be Skinny!

Mindset

Ahh! Please stop saying this, IMMEDIATELY!

The quickest way to set yourself up for failure is with a negative mindset. You could eat all the healthiest food, exercise for an hour each day, but if you're still talking down to yourself, you could be sabotaging all of your efforts and not seeing results.

You see, it is our thoughts that end up creating our reality. When we think something, we create an energetic vibration that matches the thought. Then our emotions become involved, which affect our body's chemistry, which reinforce the beliefs that we hold about something.

When we combine thoughts with emotions, we are combining an electrical force with a magnetic force, hence creating a strong electromagnetic force. This is how we create.

Everything around us is comprised of energy. When we have an electromagnetic force at work inside us, it results in us taking certain actions – engaging with our surroundings in a certain way that will ultimately produce a certain effect.

For instance, if you look in the mirror each day and tell yourself how fat you are, you are thinking this, feeling it, and as a result, causing your body to believe it. The body doesn't know the difference between real or imaginary when you produce the thoughts and emotions to support a belief, and hence, it will give you the result of these feelings. So if you constantly tell yourself you are fat, you will be fat.

On the other hand, if you look in the mirror, and tell yourself how beautiful you are; if you can visualize yourself looking and feeling exactly the way you want to – happy, light, and full of energy, this is what your body will begin to deliver to you.

It's an amazing thing how the mind works.

If you're interested in learning more about the neuroscience behind this, I highly recommend the book "Buddha's Brain" by Richard Hanson.

There are several practices we can incorporate into our daily routines to help improve our mindset so that we can reach our goals and achieve the results we are looking for. I'll list them here, and then we'll explore them each in a little more depth:

- Gratitude

- Positivity

- Visualization

Gratitude

Gratitude is the fastest way to change our external circumstances. As I mentioned earlier, what we focus our attention on is what becomes our reality.

By appreciating the little things in life, as well as the big, we start to bring our attention to all the wonderful things that are happening. The opposite holds true as well – if we focus on the negative, we end up seeing negative all around, and therefore invite and experience more negative.

When we take the time to express gratitude, it actually trains our brains to seek out the good. (It is our natural tendency to seek out the bad, as this is essential for survival, but in today's society, it is not needed as it was thousands of years ago when we were in constant danger of being attacked by predators.)

So in order to do this, we must make a conscious effort to express gratitude as much as possible, until it becomes a habit, and then a way of life.

I recommend you start your day with a few moments of gratitude. Before you get out of bed in the morning, right after you wake up, simply give thanks for the new day and you can mentally list a few of the many things you are grateful for.

At night, before you go to bed, do this practice again, this time writing them down in a journal. Try to list five things each day that you are grateful for, and make them something different each day.

You can even set yourself a reminder for a certain time during your day to express gratitude. You can use an alarm on your phone for instance. Make it your gratitude alarm, set to go off at the same time each day.

This simple practice of expressing gratitude can change your life. I encourage you to start today. Right now. This moment.

Positivity

In addition to gratitude, it's crucial to also keep a general positive mindset. As I mentioned, our thoughts are what create our reality, so we want to do our best to maintain mostly positive thoughts.

For many of us, this may be hard. However, it's not impossible. The first step in the process is awareness. By bringing awareness to the act of negative thinking, we can then begin to change it.

Let's go back to the example of looking at ourselves in the mirror. This is the perfect demonstration of how positivity can come into play. When you first catch yourself thinking something negative, simply start by bringing awareness to the fact that you are doing it.

The next step is to replace it with something positive. So as we did in the mirror example, we changed our thoughts to something positive in order to produce a more positive outcome. Now, this doesn't mean you're going to instantly shed twenty pounds as you stand in front of the mirror, but it will make it much easier for you to shed that weight over time in a healthy way.

As a culture, we are largely focused on instant gratification and seeking immediate results. This unfortunately, can lead to more fluctuation in the outcomes we produce, and more frustration.

Therefore, it's essential that we cultivate patience and consistency when we practice positivity. Conditions don't usually change overnight, especially when they've been present for a very long time. Therefore, consistency and patience will allow us to steadily come closer to our goals, and when we do reach them, to maintain them long term.

So, the next exercise I would like to offer you is one of positive affirmations. You may create a list of ten or more positive affirmations related to your specific goal (i.e. losing twenty pounds), or you may use the examples provided below:

I completely love and respect myself and my body.

My body is a gift that allows me to experience all that life has to offer.

I am grateful for all that my body does for me.

I treat my body well.

I am happy, healthy, and radiant.

I have an abundance of energy.

I choose to eat only healthy food.

I am confident in my own skin.

I make positive, healthy choices.

I nourish my mind, body and soul.

My body is healthy, my mind is healthy, my emotions are balanced, and my spirit soars.

Once you have your list, I'd like you to read it out loud each morning, preferably while looking in the mirror - each morning.

Erasing Negative Self Talk

These positive affirmations are also an excellent way to replace negative thoughts about yourself with more positive ones. As I've explained already, our thoughts create our reality, so if you constantly tell yourself the ways in which you are not good enough, that is what you're going to cultivate more of.

The way to change this is to begin by bringing awareness to when you make a negative comment, and replace it with something positive.

When we become disconnected from our bodies, we become fragmented. And that is when 'dis-ease', including weight gain, becomes a constant struggle.

There are so many different reasons why we might treat ourselves in this way – we could have had bad role models, perhaps someone constantly put us down when we were younger, maybe we were held to unrealistic standards. It could just be our own expectations that we're not meeting that are causing us to talk negatively about ourselves. Whatever the situation is for you, it's time to stop.

Goal Setting

Before we move on, I'd like to take a moment to emphasize the importance of goal setting. Now that we've cultivated a more positive mindset, it's important to define a clear and specific goal that we want to achieve.

We can ask ourselves the question: "What do I want to achieve?" Please be specific, using concrete measurables such as a number of pounds you want to lose, or a dress size you'd like to fit into. Once you have this, please write it down.

Next, we will look at the question of when, "When do I want to achieve this by?" Again, please be specific. Give yourself an exact date that you would like to have this goal accomplished. Please be realistic, but don't make it so far out that it seems like it will never come.

For example, if you're goal is to lose 40 pounds, this obviously won't happen in one week, but it doesn't need to take five years. Find the point of balance that you honestly feel you can achieve, and that will provide motivation for you to work toward. Once you have the date, go ahead and write out a full sentence for your goal and the date you would like to have it accomplished by in the format "My goal is to _____ by _____."

You can also begin with a smaller, more manageable goal, such as losing ten pounds, and set a date for that to happen. By working in smaller increments, it can help keep the motivation high as you achieve these milestones and track your progress.

By having this very specific goal and timeline in place, it will you a point of focus and direction to work toward. Having a clear goal will allow all of the supporting actions to fall into place for you to be able to reach it.

Visualization

Now that you have your goal clearly defined, it's time to set things in motion with visualization. By visualizing the outcome you want to achieve, you can train your mind and body to facilitate the progress needed to make it a reality.

As described earlier, our mind doesn't really know the difference between what is "real" and what is in our imagination. (What is actually *real* is a whole other topic that I don't have room to cover in this book, but please visit my website www.TheWisdomOfWellness.com to sign up for my newsletter if this interests you, as I will certainly address this in other writings).

I also mentioned the electromagnetic force that is created when we combine the power of our thoughts and emotions. Therefore, the process will go like this: each night, before you go to sleep, I encourage you to take a few moments to do a visualization practice. It can be right after you write in your gratitude journal. You can begin by doing the breathing exercise I outlined in the beginning of the chapter, and this time, feel free to lie down on your back if you prefer. You can do it right in your bed as long as you're not going to fall asleep during the process (if you feel like you are, it is better to sit upright).

Next, start to visualize your life as it would be once you've reached the specific goal you've set. Imagine what you would be doing, how you would be feeling, and really try to manifest the experience of being in the state.

Create the positive feelings that come along with reaching your goals, as if you've already reached them. Do this for at least five minutes, feeling, thinking, and being as if you have already reached your specific goal. See it in your mind's eye and feel it in your body and your heart.

Do this every night before you go to sleep. This practice will set you up to manifest this vision as a reality, and when done before bed, has the added bonus of working at the subconscious level while we are sleeping.

It is this subconscious level that we need to address to ultimately make a shift, as the conscious is only part of the equation.

It's Not About Being Skinny

In addition to having a clearly defined goal, it's important to understand the deeper reasons why we want to achieve it. Do you simply want to be skinny for the sake of being skinny? I doubt it. What does losing weight mean for you? Perhaps it's about having more self-confidence to do the things you want to do such as dating; perhaps it's more of a health concern so you can reverse or prevent certain conditions; or perhaps you simply want to have more energy and be able to move about more freely in your body so that you can enjoy all the fun activities you used to do or to keep up with your kids or grandkids.

Whatever it is for you, it's a good practice to identify that when you're setting your goals, and to keep it in mind as you go through your weight loss journey. If you're ever faced with a challenging situation, this can help tremendously to remind you why you are doing what you're doing and to help keep you on track.

In direct response to the idea of being "skinny", I'd like to share a story with you. When I was in my early twenties, I decided to become a raw vegan, thinking it was the healthiest way to eat. You'll find out why in a moment, but boy was I wrong!!! The things I didn't know then that Ayurveda has since taught me could have saved me a lot of hardship.

Let Go and Lose Weight

It started off great, I switched my diet all at once (as this is the way I did things back then, very extreme), and I started losing weight almost immediately. 'This is great!' I thought to myself, despite the long hours of food preparation, including soaking, sprouting, grinding, dehydrating, and so on.

Now, please keep in mind, I wasn't doing it solely to lose weight, although that was certainly part of it, but I honestly believed it was a healthy way to eat based on all the talk of enzymes being preserved when food is eaten raw, and so on. So I was off to a great start.

But sadly, my cravings for sweets did not go away as I followed this new diet; if anything, they actually became worse. So along with my green veggies, sprouted seeds, and fresh fruit, I was eating tons of dried fruit, including calorie dense dates, and others like dried pineapple, figs, etc. Now this may not seem inherently bad, but if you examined my diet, it was extremely high in sugar. This is not good.

And in addition to that, dried fruits can severely back you up if they are not soaked, and I was already prone to constipation due to my constitution. What made it even worse is that raw foods in general are difficult for the body to digest, and I was eating them in humungous portions in an attempt to get enough calories!

I would consume heaping bowls of salad and other raw veggie combinations, supplemented by snacking on lots of dried fruit (and frequent snacking is another digestive disaster, which we'll get more into later in Chapter 6), so after initially feeling a state of cleansing and release, imagine how I felt not too long after…yes, you guessed it, completely backed up and bloated!

I spent my days in so much pain!!! I was so gassy, and I wasn't having regular bowel movements, my poor little tummy was protruding like I was in my second trimester! By this point, I had lost quite a bit of weight, so the bloated tummy looked pretty extreme on me.

Not only that, but the weight I had lost included lots of lean muscle mass. I was rail-thin now (except for the bloated tummy), however, it was mostly due to the water and muscle I lost. (Yes, I lost fat too, but in the process, I lost much needed muscle).

So now here I was, nice and "skinny", but I felt like crap. I was extremely cold all the time, and my mood sunk so low, I just laid in bed, trying to get warm, when I wasn't working or preparing food. I didn't have any energy to deal with the world.

This continued for two years, yes, two years! And along the way, my hair began falling out, I had intense dark bags under my eyes (which I had never experienced before), my skin was an absolute mess, breaking out all the time, and I constantly had canker sores in my mouth due to a nutrient deficiency.

My family kept pleading with me that I was getting to thin, but I reassured them that I was eating a healthy diet of organic *raw* food and was fine.

Eventually, I began to realize how utterly awful I felt, both physically and mentally, and I also started to have extreme cravings – for sweets, for sustenance, for nourishment!

I began eating more raw nuts in an attempt to satisfy these cravings, and I saw my weight start to slowly creep up. How can anyone *gain* weight on a raw food diet!? Well, nuts are heavy and hard to digest, and my digestive fire was already ruined from the diet I'd been on, so it wasn't too far-fetched.

It wasn't until one fateful December night, as my roommate was in the process of making dozens of fabulous homemade cookies in preparation for the holidays, and I found myself secretly binging on them when she left the house, that I knew it was time for something to be done! I had no self-control; I was a complete slave to the cookies!

I would open the door to the fridge, look at them, salivate, go to the other room and think about them, until finally I caved and ate a whole bunch. She actually walked in on me because she forgot something and she started cracking up! It was the funniest thing to her because for the two years that she'd known me, I had been raw vegan the whole time, and there I was, going to town on a plate full of sugary cookies! (It is pretty funny looking back on it, but not really :p)

After much convincing from my roommate, I started with a piece of raw salmon and I can't even begin to describe what I felt when I took that first bite. A whole flood of "feel-good" chemicals started rushing through my body, and after a few bites I literally felt like I was high!

It was such an amazing feeling, and after depriving my body for so long, was exactly what it needed. I gradually made the shift into eating some cooked food on a regular basis. Why gradually when I'd jumped right into the raw vegan full-force? Because my digestive power had become so weakened by that type of diet over the past two years, that my body wasn't able to process more than a very small amount of cooked food at one time. It would be like lead in my stomach.

I was nearly heartbroken – the raw food made me terribly bloated and gassy, and the cooked food sat in my stomach like a rock. What was I supposed to do??

Luckily, my digestive fire (known as *agni* in Ayurveda) gradually began to strengthen until I was able to digest complete meals again. (Just to note however, besides the fish, I maintained an otherwise "vegan" diet for some time after that).

It wasn't until a few years later, when I began practicing Ayurveda, that I would discover the extent to which I had damaged my *agni*. With raw foods being so difficult to digest, except for those with the strongest of pitta constitutions (pitta being made up of the fire element, which we'll get into more later), it is important to dress them with plenty of healthy fats and digestive spices to aid in digestion and absorption. And, for someone who has a good deal of vata (air and space elements) in their constitution, as I do, it should never comprise the majority of our meals.

This was completely contradictory to what I was doing with my raw food diet. It wasn't the majority of my meals, it *was* my meals! And I didn't know anything about digestive spices back then. No wonder I experienced so much gas and bloating! (Not to mention terrible constipation).

It took me nearly two years after practicing Ayurveda to restore my digestive fire to an optimum state. Not that I didn't see improvement sooner, but to reach its *optimum state*.

Having experienced this is why I always encourage my clients to have patience and be consistent. It may sound discouraging that something took that long to regain its full capacity, but we must consider the time that went into throwing it out of balance prior to that.

And I can almost assure you that I did not have optimally functioning digestive capacity before my raw vegan years, so it was likely many, many years of poor and incorrect eating habits that had weakened my digestive fire, and the raw food experience just really put it over the edge.

Considering all that, I don't think two years sounds long at all! Fortunately, I am happy to report that after rebalancing my agni, it has been functioning quite optimally ever since ☺

One of the main points I wanted to express through this story, is that being 'skinny' is overrated. Skinny does not equal healthy, as my story demonstrated, and it certainly doesn't equal happy!

Rather, a healthy, balanced state of being can bring health and happiness – in mind, body, heart and soul.

Chapter Three | Toxic Belief # 3: Every Time I Try To Lose Weight I Feel Deprived – It's Not Worth It!

It's Not About Deprivation

Let me start by emphasizing this – losing weight is not about deprivation! I know there is a commonly held misbelief that we need to deprive ourselves in order to lose weight, but I'm here to tell you that it just ain't true! Deprivation can work temporarily, but while also making you miserable - but who wants to live a life in misery??

I remember when I was in college, I got into a very strict fitness routine, I was going to the gym for a couple of hours a day – lifting weights, running, etc. I was in amazing physical shape. I became so focused on perfecting my physique that I strictly limited my food intake, actually counting out a specific number of almonds to have as a snack (I think it was 12 raw almonds), and weighing and measuring every single portion of food that I ate. I would not allow myself any "cheat" foods, and if I did splurge and had a few organic corn tortilla chips, I would be able to tell the next day how it affected me.

I was so strict with my eating, however, I was not getting enough calories in relation to the amount of physical activity I was doing. I was following some guidelines I had read in a women's fitness magazine, not taking into account the fact that **we are all unique individuals**.

This one-size-fits-all approach did not work well for me, as I'm sure it doesn't work well for most people. I remember buying a bar of organic dark chocolate, and storing it on the shelf in my closet. Whenever I had the craving for it, I would open the door and look at it, but I would never eat it. Somehow, knowing it was there made me feel better, crazy as it may be.

Needless to say, this approach did not last long - I was always starving, and always miserable, and that is no way to live!

Food and Pleasure

Eating is one of the essential aspects of survival, and a big part of being human! So why would we want to deprive ourselves of enjoying this experience?

Rather than looking at eating as something that makes you put on weight, I encourage you to look at it from a new perspective – a more sacred perspective.

You see, in my view, everything is divine. You are divine, I am divine, and the food we eat is divine. Every morsel of food that I put into my mouth I now see as a blessing. It sustains me and nourishes me so that I can continue to do good work in the world.

When we change our viewpoint and begin to look at eating from this new view, it can completely change the effect that the food has on us! And not only does food nourish on the physical level, but it can nourish on all levels, including the emotional and mental.

I'm sure you've heard of how certain foods are good for your brain, or can boost mood – this is just an example of how food nourishes us a whole beings, not just a body looking to reduce mass.

As we discovered in the first chapter, our mindset is everything. It determines our success and our failure, more than you may realize. Since it is the factor driving our experience of 'reality', why not take the reins and create what you want?

To this end, it's important that we enjoy our food and find it appealing on multiple sensory levels – it should be visually appealing, it should smell good, taste good, and the texture should feel good to us. If we try to limit ourselves to bland "diet" food, our bodies will not be getting what they need, and we will end up having cravings.

Your body is intelligent! If you are depriving it of something essential, healthy fats for instance, it will start to crave these things in an effort to balance itself out. So the quickest way to fail at weight loss is to eat bland, tasteless food that is unappealing.

Therefore, it's important to learn how to prepare your food in such a manner that it can still be healthy, but also taste good at the same time. In Ayurveda, oils such as ghee (clarified butter) and coconut oil are used, along with a variety of spices. Not only do these aid in digestion and assimilation, but they also help prevent the food from tasting bland.

Thinking back to my college days again, I remember eating grilled chicken, steamed broccoli, and rice, all measured out in exact proportions, and all bland as heck! I had no clue about how to make food taste good while keeping it healthy. I hardly used any spices in my cooking, and I didn't even know how to make the rice taste good, it was awful! Perhaps if I'd had some better exposure to healthy cooking methods, I would have enjoyed my meals more.

To get you started with some amazing Ayurvedic recipes, I highly recommend the cookbook *Heaven's Banquet*. It's a compilation of recipes from around the world, adjusted to meet Ayurvedic cooking guidelines. These recipes are not complicated, and they're absolutely delicious! I gift a copy to all of my clients when they start a program with me, and you can find it right on Amazon. It's a great resource; I recommend you check it out.

Cooking as Sadhana

The term *sadhana* refers to a daily spiritual practice. I would like to introduce to you the idea of cooking as a spiritual practice. As we know that eating is essential to our survival and proper nourishment, I feel that cooking certainly should be a spiritual practice.

As you consider the different levels of human experience: the physical, energetic, emotional, mental and spiritual, you see that they are all intimately connected. What happens to one will eventually feed up or down into the others.

So if we maintain good nutrition, it can indeed affect our mental and emotional health, as science has proven, and it can also affect our spiritual well-being. And for a truly balanced and fulfilling life, we must address all of these areas, not just one or two.

Working in the other direction, as we cultivate more time for spirituality, it can start to affect our mental health and our emotional health, which can then, through the energetic body, feed into our physical health. So observing cooking as a spiritual practice can immediately benefit us on the higher level of spirituality, as well as the gross level of physicality. The benefits of both, flowing into each other and sustaining all the other levels while doing so.

What are a few ways that we can begin to create this practice? Well, these days, I know a lot of my clients feel rushed in their lives, as do many of us. There are so many responsibilities, so many hats to wear, so much to get done in the mere twenty-four hours of our day. Often, they will relegate cooking to be an inconvenient chore. This, unfortunately, is only going to work to their detriment.

When we eat food that is processed, pre-prepared, or micro-waved, we miss out on the vital life force energy known as *prana*. And with the loss of *prana*, we also lose out on vitamins, nutrients, and other essential components. At this point, the food becomes more like dead mass we ingest in order to quell a rumbling tummy, rather than nourishment.

To visualize this a little better, take a moment to picture your body in your mind's eye. (After you read this section you can take a moment to close your eyes if you'd like). See your body as the living, thriving organism that it is. Teeming with life – the blood flowing, the energy pulsating; your heart beats, your lungs breath, and juices move through your stomach and intestines; not to mention all the activity that is going on in your brain! There is so much at work here, so much going on and so much life to be had.

Now, imagine a fresh, juicy piece of fruit, just picked from the tree. It is ripe with life, full of color and water, vitamins and nutrients from the sun that is shining on it, the soil and the tree. And since it was just picked, it is still full of *prana*, that vital life force energy. Now, imagine ingesting this delicious, juicy piece of fruit, with all the goodness it has to offer. All of this goodness becomes a part of you as your body happily accepts the offering, digests it and assimilates the nutrients into your body. The *prana* then adds to *your* prana, causing you to feel nourished, full of life and energy. Since it is so well liked by your body, it is digested and processed easily and efficiently.

Now I would like you to consider another scenario. Think about this same piece of delicious fruit, however, this time, imagine it was picked before it was fully ripe, and then left to sit in a dark crate while it's transported across the country. After that, it sits on a shelf for some time before you find it and pick it up. You then take it home and put it on one of *your* shelves for a few more days before finally eating it.

By this point, the fruit is no longer juicy, it is pretty dried up actually, it does not have the bright, bold color or ripeness, it is more pale and lacking, and you can tell when you bite into it that it does not have much flavor. It's a little harder to chew, and not that satisfying. Please take a moment to consider the different way your body will react to this piece of fruit vs. the fresh, juicy, ripe piece.

Now, I would like you to take it one step further. This time, instead of imagining a piece of fruit, I would like you to imagine you are at the grocery store and you pick up a frozen 'diet' dinner. You look at the ingredients, and everything is organic, but there are still some items on the list you cannot pronounce. You take it home and pop it in the microwave while you catch up on some chores.

When you go to eat it, how do you feel? How much life force do you think is left in there after it's been 1) processed, 2) frozen, and 3) zapped by microwave radiation? This 'food' is not fresh; it likely has no vital life force left at that point. I hesitate to even call it 'food' anymore. On top of this, what are those chemicals that were added to preserve it, and how does your body react to them? (I'll tell you how very quickly, in case you're not aware – your body may see them as a foreign invader and try to attack it with the immune system; it may also begin to create fat around your vital organs in order to protect them from the toxicity. The body is intelligent, it will act to defend itself, and this is how).

How much nutrition do you think you will actually get by consuming this 'dead' food? Not much. And, it's likely causing your body to store fat in order to protect itself. (Your body creates fat around your organs to protect them from toxic invaders).

So, now that your body in malnourished, what will it do? Well, it will likely cause you to have cravings, because it is still looking for the nourishment it hasn't received. Meanwhile, that dead matter you ingested is having a difficult time making its way through your system, as your body is so confused and doesn't know what to do with it. As a result, you might suffer from constipation.

This does not sound like the situation I would want to be in; I'll stick with the fresh piece of fruit, thank you!

Now, I'm not saying you have to survive off of fruit alone to maintain your weight, the point of this exercise was to get you to see the difference between food that is fresh, and foo that is not, and the different effects it can have on your physiology. We didn't even get into the effects on our mental and emotional health that can be caused by eating stale and processed foods, but they are just as bad.

The top five qualities you'll want to look for in the food you eat include:

1. Fresh

2. Local

3. Organic (Biodynamic is even better)

4. Unprocessed

5. Not microwaved or overcooked

Slowing It Down

Now that we've covered the basics of what quality of foods to eat, it's important to mention that setting aside time to prepare and consume the food is essential.

Most of us rush through our days and our meals, but when we do this, the food isn't as nourishing, and it's not digested as well. So by making food prep and mealtime a priority, we can come closer to our weight loss goals. Some other tips to keep in mind:

- Try to give your full attention to the food as you are preparing and eating it

- Avoid distractions such as television, working, driving, etc. while eating

- Aim to eat in a calm, settled environment; being under stress while eating significantly reduces our digestive ability

- Chew your food thoroughly; enjoy the taste, texture and experience while eating

- Tune into your stomach as you're eating, let it guide you as to when it's had enough; this is usually *before* you feel full

The Energetics of Food

Another important point to consider is the energetics going *into* the food you consume. If you're new to the concept of other people's energy affecting things around them, consider this scenario – your partner comes home from work, and they just had a heated argument with their boss. They are upset due to this, and very tense. Although they don't come out and say anything right away, you can *feel* it, and know they are experiencing some type of upset.

This is just a very basic example, but energy affects those around us on a much more subtle level as well. In this section, I'll be focusing on it specifically as it relates to food. Do you remember your grandma cooking for you as a child, and how absolutely amazing everything tasted? It was likely because she put so much love into it!

The opposite holds true as well – if someone is experiencing mental stress or tensions while they're preparing your food, that energy is being transmitted into the meal, and then you will be taking that in when you consume it. Who wants that!? Not I.

This is why it's important to cook your own food as much as possible. When you go out to a restaurant, besides not knowing all the ingredients and preparation methods used (very often then use microwaves to reheat and cook with low quality oils), you don't know what kind of mood the cooks are in. If they're feeling stressed out and overwhelmed at work, that's the type of energy that is going into your food that you'll be taking in. If they're feeling downright angry, that's what you'll get too!

Not to say that you should never eat out, but I would recommend sticking to places where you know the staff and how they are treated, as well as their cooking methods and ingredients. If there's a local food store or café that you know follows best practices, it's great to frequent these types of places when eating out.

I'm lucky – where I live, we have a small organic café and I know the owner as well as the staff, and before I ever ate there, I asked them questions about their food prep, including whether they use fresh beans that they soak, or canned beans. To might delight, everything is made fresh, and they don't even have a microwave on site!

There is also a food co-op right down the road from me, and the kitchen space is out in the open, so you can see the actual food as it's being prepared. Again, everything is made fresh daily, down to the stock for the soups! It's all organic and biodynamic, and the ingredients for all the prepared dishes are clearly listed. These are places I can feel good about eating at, so I recommend you explore what is available near you. If nothing, perhaps you can start a weekly potluck with friend and others in the neighborhood, be creative!

When you do find yourself at a restaurant, feel free to strike up a conversation with the cooks and staff; they're usually more than happy to talk to you. And a tip for when you're eating at a restaurant – don't be afraid to ask for substitutions. For example, I will ask for my food to be prepared with butter instead of oil, as I know most places use very low quality cooking oils in order to keep costs down. (Oils are one of the foods that have the most profound impact on our physiology, along with animal products, so it's important to stick to high quality). Any decent restaurant will be happy to oblige to keep their customers satisfied and coming back. So please don't be afraid to speak up.

One more area to address is the energetics in the animal products you consume, if you chose to consume these. Commercial methods for meat production are pretty harsh to say the least. I'm not going to get into too much detail here, as I don't want to be too graphic, but suffice it to say that the conditions the animals have to endure are nothing less than heart breaking.

The method in which they are slaughtered also adds an element of fear, and the animals bodies produce a flood of stress hormones, including cortisol, which are then infused within their meat when you consume it. This is what you're taking into your body. You are what you eat; it's as simple as that. If you eat something that is loaded with stress hormones, they're not going to simply dissipate without having any effect on you as you ingest it.

If you chose to eat animal products, I highly, highly recommend sticking to those from local farms whenever possible; that were humanely raised, and follow organic practices or better. Grass-fed, free roaming, and with no antibiotics or hormones administered. (The same concept applies to antibiotics and hormones, if the animal ingests these, and you ingest the animals' meat, you are ingesting the same things that they did. This leads to antibiotic resistance and also weight gain from growth hormones that are used to fatten the animals).

So in addition to cooking at home, and sticking to food sources that we can feel good about by knowing their sourcing and cooking methods, how else can we raise the levels of positive energy that are in our food? Well, what I like to do it to say a prayer, or sing something uplifting while cooking. This raises my energetic vibration, which then translates into the food I'm preparing. I also like to express gratitude or say a prayer right before eating.

Finally, if I feel like the food needs a little "boost", I will hover my hands over it and send all the positive, loving vibrations that I can toward it. Again, if the concept of moving energy is new to you, it may seem a little hard to grasp, but consider these facts given to us by the study of physics in that everything is made up of vibrating particles of energy, and according to the First Law of Thermodynamics:

- Energy cannot be created or destroyed, but it can change form

Please consider this for a moment in relation to the key points we've address above – transfer of energy from person to food, to person and transfer of energy from animal to person. With the scientific backup supporting the transformation of energy, why should the concepts I've presented seem so outrageous? It is only in our limited thinking that things seem impossible. As you allow your mind to become more expansive, new worlds will open up to you.

Redefining That Which Satisfies

Currently, you may associate certain foods as tasting "good" to you, such as heavy, oily, sweet, or processed foods, and not be able to imagine giving these up.

Fortunately, I have good news. As you begin to clean up your diet and eat more wholesome foods, your taste preferences will begin to change. The foods that once tasted so savory and delicious will no longer have the same effect. The cleaner you start to eat, the less unwholesome foods you will crave.

Many foods, such as sugar and those with chemical additives, have an addictive effect as well, working on our brain's chemistry to keep us wanting more. As you wean yourself off of these, they too will no longer have the same hold on you. As a result, you will find it easier to stay on a clean eating routine as you nourish and balance your body through proper nutrition.

I've experienced this first hand. I used to have the worst sugar addiction! I would crave sweets constantly. These days, I can't have anything with much sugar at all, else it feels way too overwhelming to me, and not enjoyable in the least. If I do have something that is sweet, I immediately feel like I need to brush my teeth as it becomes that overpowering.

A good tip for working through this process or for times when you slip up, is to sip a cup of hot water after you ate the offending food. It will help it to be digested better so that it moves through your system quicker and more efficiently, thus avoiding overwhelming toxic build up.

It brings a deep sense of freedom to not be addicted to sugar anymore. And with the reduction of sugar in my diet comes the added benefits of increased energy due to more stable blood sugar levels; a more balanced mood also due to less variation in blood sugar levels; better sleep, and improved immune function.

I don't even want to get into processed foods – if I ever try to eat something "artificial", it tastes absolutely disgusting to me. (I've done tests to try it out – at parties where all sorts of concoctions are being served). I don't make it a regular habit, but from time to time I get curios and put a little in my mouth, and I can literally feel the film of chemical residue on my tongue. I usually end up spitting it out.

The look of these foods doesn't even entice me anymore. I remember years ago, seeing all the wonderful sweets piled up on the table at Christmas dinner used to drive me out of my mind! My mouth would water at the sight of them. Nowadays, it all just looks like dry, processed flour and chemicals, which has no appeal to me.

So if you struggle with food addictions, I hope this can serve as inspiration, know that it can be overcome! I was a huge sugar addict and now I am free from its pull.

In addition, as you start to clean up your diet, you will start to feel better physically, emotionally, and mentally. When all of these areas become more balanced, food will no longer have the same hold over you. And as you're working through the process, you can always think back to how you felt before you improved your diet, and it can serve as motivation to stay on the right path.

Keeping a journal can be a useful practice to help you track how you feel along your journey. You'll be able to look back and see all the progress you've made along the way, and this can serve as ongoing motivation and inspiration for you. I recommend writing down specific things you can measure, such as how you feel when you wake up in the morning, your average energy levels during the day on a scale from 1 – 10, and so on. Sometimes, once you start feeling so good and just pop out of bed with no problem, and fly through your day full of energy and clarity, you can forget how bad you felt before! So in times when you might be thinking about veering off this new path, journaling can be a very useful tool.

Symptoms such as brain fog, low energy, digestive disturbances, headaches, acne, and more, can start to clear up as you improve our diet. Once you feel the lightness and freedom in your body, you will never want to go back! Proper nutrition also helps to stabilize your hormones and mood, all very positive benefits to look forward to.

Please remember however, that these can be the results when you eat in a balanced way, not an extreme way. So if you've "dieted" in the past, and felt really crappy, try not to associate that with eating a "healthy diet". A healthy diet, as we already discussed, is not about deprivation or lack. It is about good nutrition, good preparation, and satisfaction. This approach will help you to achieve and maintain your goals long term.

Chapter Four | Toxic Belief # 4: I Don't Have the Energy to Exercise, and Even If I Wanted to, There Is No Time

I understand how difficult it can be to find the motivation to exercise when you are completely exhausted, but as we begin to explore this further, you will see how regular exercise can actually help to *increase* your energy levels.

There are a few ways it does this, including: 1) Improving the quality of your sleep, 2) Improving circulation, and 3) Decreasing your natural stress response, all of which serve to naturally increase your energy levels.

The Importance of Proper Sleep and The Stress Response

Not only can insufficient or poor quality sleep leave you feeling exhausted, it can also put you at greater risk for a number of illnesses including heart disease, diabetes, weight gain, and more. The reason it sets you up for weight gain, is that it activates the sympathetic nervous system, producing the "fight or flight" response. This sets off a series of reactions in your body, including the release of stress hormones, such as cortisol.

This entire process affects the gastrointestinal system, leading to an impaired ability to digest food and eliminate waste. Cortisol can also lead to visceral fat storage, better known as belly fat.

In addition, when you are tired, you may crave sweets in the body's attempt to procure energy, and you may also feel more hungry, as it disrupts your appetite signals. When you're exhausted from insufficient sleep, you are also less likely to have the energy and motivation to do things like exercise, prepare health meals, and so on.

Poor sleep can also affect your mood, making it even harder for you to stick with healthy lifestyle choices. The effects are detrimental to your health.

One of the best things you can do to help improve your sleep is to get regular exercise. Regular movement can help you to not only fall asleep easier, but to also have better quality sleep.

A few tips to incorporating exercise if you are chronically tired:

- Start with something gentle, such as a walk or stretching.

- Think about what time of day you have the most energy, it might be in the morning, or right before lunch, and make an effort to schedule your exercise for this time. It may seem like a challenge if you have a very busy schedule, but by putting it in your calendar and treating it with the importance it deserves, it will become doable. It all comes down to prioritizing that which is important to us.

- Try to do something you find enjoyable, such as a team sport or anything else you can look forward to. Usually, once you start moving, your energy levels may start to increase immediately, giving you the ability to keep going.

Exercise and The Chakra System

From a yogic perspective, exercise can directly affect they chakra system. Chakras are described as vital energy centers that run along the spine. There are seven main chakras that form the basis of this system, each representing a different aspect of our mental/emotional experience. Below is a brief summary of each, beginning from the base of the spine up:

1. **Muladhara** – the root chakra, or 1st chakra, located at the base of the spine, at about the level of the coccyx bone, is said to represent that which is related to survival.

2. **Swadhisthana** – located at the level of the lower abdomen, a couple of inches below the belly button, is said to represent our emotions and sexuality.

3. **Manipura** – located at the solar plexus, is said to represent our self-identification, including our self-esteem and will power.

4. **Anahata** – located at the heart, is said to represent our capacity for love and compassion, as well as self-acceptance and acceptance of others.

5. **Vissudha** – located at the throat, it represents our capacity for self-expression and speaking one's truth.

6. **Ajna** – the third eye chakra, located between the eyebrows and about two finger widths up; represents our intuition.

7. **Sahasrara** – the crown chakra, located at the crown of the head; representing our connection to the divine.

Certain forms of movement, such as conscious dance, can help balance the chakras; martial arts can as well. Yoga is designed to balance all the chakras, and there are specific postures that are especially good for individual chakras. Through the movements of twisting, compressing, back bending, and so forth, energetics blocks can be released, and energy can be brought to areas that are lacking.

It's a beautiful form of healing and excellent demonstration of how we can work at the physical level to create profound transformation on all levels. Starting a yoga practice completely changed my life. In brought me to a greater sense of connection with my body, and I was able to find love and respect for it like I never had before.

It also gave me a deep awareness for my body in space, including how it interacted with those around me. I think before we can become truly aware of how we affect others, we must first understand how we affect ourselves. Yoga is an excellent tool for this.

In addition to the energetic blocks it can help remove, yoga asana also makes a profound impact on the physiology and can lead to weight loss. Postures which involve twisting and compression are absolutely amazing for strengthening and regulating the entire gastro-intestinal system.

This can help regulate metabolism and allow you to burn food more efficiently. It can also help with symptoms of constipation, gas, and other discomforts. By optimizing your body's ability to digest food and eliminate waste, you set yourself up to release excess weight naturally.

Other postures, such as inversions, are excellent for promoting circulation, and stimulating important parts of the brain, such as the pituitary gland, which help to decrease your stress response and regulate mood.

Another huge benefit I found from yoga was the ability to for once be able to calm and steady my mind. Prior to taking up a yoga practice, my brain was so scattered! I had constant worries running through my head, anxieties, tensions, you name it. I worried about work, I worried about life, relationships, etc.; I was never in the present moment. What I didn't realize at that time was that this tendency was a huge part of my own suffering.

By learning to meditate through movement, I finally found some peace. And just a note on meditation, in case that word scares you – it doesn't have to be anything extreme such as sitting in an uncomfortable cross legged position for a long time and thinking about nothing. It's simply learning to harness and focus your mind.

Hopefully, you can now see how a simple "exercise" can have a deeply profound impact on your body, heart, mind and soul. No longer is it just a form of movement, but it can transform into a deeply spiritual practice. By learning to be present, connect with yourself on all levels, and connect with the people and environment around you, you can find wholeness, the lack of which is often a huge driver behind habits that lead to weight gain.

Resistance Training

This is not a book on exercise, so I'm not going to go into specific detail here, but I would like to speak a little about resistance training, especially since the goal of this book is to help you lose weight.

I mentioned how I use to pretty much be a "gym rat" back in my college days, and it was quite useful during my college studies, because all of the physical activity I did really optimized by brain functioning and allowed me to achieve peak mental performance. (I'll get into that more in the following section). But what it also did was set me up with a good foundation for later in life.

Resistance training is important for many reasons. One is that is protects the body from injury. I've had personal experience with this on several occasions. Once was when I'd went off of my resistance training routine for a while, and ended up pulling my hamstring during a roundhouse kick in martial arts class.

For three years, I kept stretching the area in an attempt to alleviate the pain, not realizing that I was only making it worse! I had gone to an orthopedist at the initial onset of the injury, and his advice was rest it and I could have a steroid injection for the pain. I chose to opt-out of the injection, and instead I refrained from activity for a while to allow it to heal. But I continued to have pain for years after.

It wasn't until I began working with a corrective exercise specialist years later that I realized I needed to re-strengthen the area, and once I did, the pain finally subsided.

Now, you may be thinking to yourself "Well, I don't do martial arts, so I'll be fine". But this is just an example. Injuries can happen during everyday activities if the body is not properly conditioned, or if we are not using good form when we move, not just during extreme sports.

My second experience with this is that I used to get a lot of lower back pain, especially when I sat at a desk all day. What happens when we sit at a desk and don't condition our body is that very often, the body is prone to poor posture. The shoulders start to round, and our back slumps. Also our neck might protrude forward as we stare at the computer screen. This can leads to all sorts of aches and pains! Not only in the low back, but also the upper back, neck, and shoulders. And if you have an impingement in any of these areas, it can send nerve pain to other parts of your body including your arms, legs, glute and hip area, etc.

Resistance training can help keep the muscles of the back, shoulder, glutes, and abdominals strong, so that we can more easily hold ourselves upright. I personally do resistant training for my neck as well in order to keep my head over my shoulders, which is so important. I used to get terrible pain in my upper back, neck, and shoulders, and this resolved it.

I was so inspired by what I learned through working with the corrective exercise specialist, that I decided to get my certification as a personal trainer and then further specialize in corrective exercise. This has come in extremely helpful in my practice, as many of my clients often complain to me of these types of symptoms, and now I am able to offer sound advice to them for how to correct it.

In addition to help keeping you pain and injury free, resistance training is one of the fastest ways to burn fat! When you have more lean muscle mass, it raises your base metabolism, and helps you to more efficiently burn fat. I know a lot of women who are thin, but still complain about issues such as feeling flabby or having cellulite in certain areas. Resistance training is the answer to that.

There are so many pills, lotions, and other devices, not to mention even more expense treatments such as laser, that promise to remove cellulite. Unfortunately, these are not viable solutions, as they are not addressing the actual cause of the cellulite. All it takes is some clean eating and a few simple exercises. I wish this information was more readily available so women can stop struggling and stop wasting money on products that don't work! Hopefully this book will help spread the word. ☺

So if you are looking for a sleek, sexy physique, I highly recommend adding resistance training to your routine. You don't have to join a gym or work with a personal trainer, although, if you are new to it, I would recommend working with a trainer at first to ensure you are doing the exercises correctly and have proper form. Trainers can also be great motivators if you do not possess the drive to do it on your own.

If you do have experience with proper technique, you can invest in a few pieces of equipment such as dumbbells, to have at home. There are other items I like to use as well, including ankle weights and medicine balls, but these are not required. It just adds variety and allows you to explore different movements.

You don't even have to buy dumbbells if you don't want to. There are many exercises that can be performed using your own body weight. This may sound easy, but let me tell you, these can often be the most difficult! When done correctly, body-weight exercises are extremely challenging and effective. And if you're anything like me, you love a challenge ;-)

The variety makes things fun, and it's good to be able to explore different options and techniques to see what resonates most with you. Visit my website to learn about my favorite resources: www.TheWisdomOfWellness.com/Resources.

Aerobic Conditioning

I personally love and have a dee p respect for cardiovascular exercise, not just because of the positive effects I see in my physiology, but more importantly, from the way it boosts my mood like nothing else.

If you've ever been an avid runner, then I'm sure you're familiar with the term "runners high". In case you're not familiar, allow me to explain. What happens when we perform aerobic exercise is the brain begins to balance our levels of neurotransmitters, such as serotonin, norepinephrine, and dopamine, which lead to improved mood, and even the feeling of being in an elated state, hence the term runners high. There are other factors that build into the equation as well, however, I will avoid going into much detail for the purposes of this book.

As you focus on your activity and let your mind take a break from all the other chatter, you can also enter a highly meditative state, which is deeply healing. Aerobic exercise can help to strengthen our ability to manage stress, improve our brain functioning, leading to increased focus and memory, and help alleviate common mood disorders such as anxiety and depression.

There is too much amazing information on this topic to cover here, but if you are interested in learning more, I highly recommend the book *Spark*, by John J. Ratey, MD. In it, he talks about the connection between exercise and the brain, and the profound transformations in can bring about.

Now, I'm not suggesting you have to go out and take up a running routine to get these benefits, there are other things you can do. In fact, I caution against running on pavement, as it is not good for the joints. I personally like to go trail running when I can find a good trail (beware of branches!).

Brisk walking is a great alternative, or even more fun is dance. Dance can be profoundly healing on many levels, and you don't even have to be good. Just turn up the music in your living room, get in front of a mirror (optional), and rock it out! I love to do this several times a week.

Especially if you need an instant mood boost, not only will the movement do that for you, but if you chose the mirror option and make some funny faces at yourself while you bust a move, you may end up rolling on the floor laughing before the song is over ☺ Allowing the music to move you is a great technique to help get you going if you feel low on energy. Even better is to grab a partner!

When It Becomes Too Much

Although it's most common that most people don't get enough exercise, there are cases where people can be over-exercising. And I wanted to address that here in case it pertains to you.

I've had several clients come to me looking to lose weight, and they were so perplexed as to why they were exercising so much and eating so little, but still weren't losing any weight. There are several reasons for this, but for now I'll focus on the issue of over-exercising.

If we exercise for more than 45 minutes at a high intensity, they body begins to create free radicals, which are counter-productive to the whole point of exercising, which is to improve one's physical condition.

In addition, if you consistently over-exercise, the body can become tight and tense, and the nervous system over-stimulated, leading to being in a chronic state of stress. As we'll discuss in Chapter 6, this is a major factor that prevents us from losing weight.

So to keep it simple, a balanced exercise program is key to attaining health and weight loss. Nothing in extreme is good for you, and that applies to physical activity as well. Aim to get some form of movement every day, but you don't have to push yourself to your limit each time.

A general rule given in the teachings of Ayurveda, is that a thin layer of sweat on the forehead is healthy. If you are sweating profusely or are constantly out of breath, you've probably taken it too far.

A balanced exercise routine should add to your energy levels, not deplete them. Some soreness the following days due to lactic acid build up is normal, but if your muscles are chronically sore and you don't take time off, it's probably wise to scale back.

Other signs of overtraining include constant fatigue, loss of motivation, and injuries such as shin splints.

PART II: THE TOXIC HABITS

Chapter Five | Toxic Habit # 1: Not Preparing In Advance

Sticking to a healthy routine is all about advance planning. Although it may take some additional time at the onset, you will everntually find your rhythm and end up saving time overall. In this chapter, I'm going to share some time-saving tips and tricks with you to help accelerate the learning curve.

Planning For Success

There are some common habits of the most highly successful people in life. One of these that I've found very effective, is to plan at night for the next day. In the context of weight loss, this can include writing down what you will eat, when you will exercise, when you will meditate, etc.

By making these plans in advance, you won't be left wondering when you will get to things the next day. Especially with the busy lives most people lead these days, it's more important than ever to prioritize and schedule, less you get swept away by something else that arises and never end up putting in the time or attention that our health deserves.

Planning your meals is crucial, especially if you work outside the home. And don't just plan breakfast and lunch, make a plan for dinner as well, so that you don't find yourself in a predicament when the evening comes. Some dinners can be prepped in the morning using a slow cooker, so you'll want to make sure you have the ingredients ready in the morning.

You can prep some ingredients for your meals the night before, such as washing and chopping veggies (although freshly chopped veggies are ideal, if your schedule is more flexible at night than in the morning, it's better to do it ahead of time so that it gets done). You can organize everything into containers so that in the morning, you can just reach in and start cooking.

You can also set out any spices and cooking utensils that you'll need to use so that they are readily accessible.

Another tip is to put the slow cooker on at night, and in the morning you'll have a fresh, hot meal to take with you for lunch. You can put your food in a wide-mouth thermos so it stays warm until it's time to eat.

Alternatively, you can start something cooking on the stove in the morning, such as lentils and rice, and after ten minutes or so, transfer it to your thermos and seal it up – it will finish the cooking process inside.

I like to get my food on the stove first thing in the morning, that way it cooks while I get myself ready. Then right before I'm ready to leave, I simply transfer it to my thermos. A one-pot meal is always super convenient. You can start with your grains and protein, and then toss veggies in toward the end.

You can do the same thing with breakfast if you're not ready to eat that early, but want to take it with you. A nice pot of warm grains cooked with some nuts and spices is a hearty meal you can take with you to go in your thermos – and it definitely beats grabbing a sugary, processed cereal bar!

You can do the same with stewed fruit, or even scrambled eggs with veggies. A warm, fresh meal is never far away when you plan in advance.

Planning your meals like this will also save you precious time during the day, freeing you up for other things, such as a nice walk. It can also prevent the dreaded "I'm starving and I don't know what to eat!" which can so often end up in poor food selection as we reach for something fast and convenient.

If you'll be away from the house, make sure to take some extra food with you, just in case you need more than anticipated. Some fresh fruit, nuts, or seeds are always a great, portable option. For variety, you can find pumpkin and sunflower seeds that have been doused with delicious spices at the health food store or online. I recently came upon an Ayurvedic seed blend! It was fantastic.

In addition to planning your food prep, it's important to also plan your shopping trips. Don't wait until the last minute when you are out of something and have no time to go to the store. As I prefer my food as fresh as possible, I prefer not to just go shopping once a week, but I certainly don't want to spend all my free time running to the grocery store.

What I do instead, is plan out when I will be near different stores so that I can stop by when I'm in the area or passing by. Where I live, there are a number of health food stores in the surrounding towns. So I will make a note of which day I will be in which area so I can visit each of them.

In addition to making shopping more convenient by planning this way, there are a couple of other reasons why it's beneficial to shop at more than one store:

1. **Variety** – by shopping at different stores, you have access to a wider variety of items such as fresh produce. If you know that one store procures locally-sourced products, you can plan to get those items there.

2. **Access to unique items**- some items, such as your favorite brand of coconut oil, might not be available at every store. In knowing where they are available, you'll be able to restock before you run out.

3. **Price** – as you shop at different stores, you'll get to know the prices for certain items vs. at other stores. It always amazes me how some stores have better prices on certain items, but not as good on others. This allows me to plan my shopping accordingly and can add up to big savings over time!

Shopping and cooking don't have to feel like chores if we plan in advance. With a little strategic thinking, we can integrate them seamlessly into our day.

And the benefits definitely outweigh the costs – you will be less likely to make poor food choices due to being caught in a pinch; you'll be able to keep a full stock of the freshest foods at the best available prices; and you'll always have a delicious, home-cooked meal available, even if you're not home when you eat it.

Eating Out

I get a lot of questions from clients about what to do when eating out, so I want to take some time to address that here. I already mentioned it in a previous chapter, and recommended looking for healthy places to eat, and making special requests when ordering. But I know that sometimes, the choice of venue is not within our control, especially if we have to go to a business dinner, or other event.

In these cases, I have a few additional tips to help.

- Avoid heavy sauces, or any sauce that sounds suspicious (ie, containing chemical additives). Instead, ask for your food to be prepared without the sauce, and substitute it with some fresh butter or olive oil and some spices or fresh herbs.

- Always ask how the food is prepared. If it's deep fried, or fried over a very high heat, ask if you can have it steam or baked instead. Most oils cannot withstand very high heat and they become carcinogenic, so it's best to avoid high-temperature cooking methods.

- If something comes breaded, ask if you can have it without the breadcrumbs.

- Avoid combining meat or eggs with dairy, it is not a good food combination and can lead to toxic buildup in the body. I know a lot of menu items at restaurants combine either meet or eggs with dairy products (think cheese, butter, yogurt, cream, etc.), so be sure to ask for it without the dairy, or chose something else.

- Skip dessert. I know this may be hard at first, but most restaurants serve desserts made with processed white flour and sugar. This just becomes sludge in our digestive tract, and can impede the digestion of our meal, leading to symptoms of indigestion. Don't opt for the fruit thinking it's healthier – fruit should always be eaten *before* other food, not after, as it can lead to poor digestion, gas, bloating, and toxic buildup when eaten after a meal.

- Skip the bread. It's unnecessary.

- Avoid sugary beverages such as iced tea, soda drinks, and fruit juices (especially fruity alcohol drinks). They add extra sugar and empty calories and can negatively affect digestion.

- Avoid ice water. It seriously impedes digestion. Instead, ask for a cup of hot water.

- Avoid sparkling water. The carbonation can lead to gas and bloating.

- Bring your own *churna* (spice mix) with you in a little jar. Sprinkle it on all of your food to aid digestion and assimilation. Some of my clients tell me they feel self-conscious doing this. My advice – get over it! Who cares what anyone else thinks? It's your health, not theirs.

- Try to avoid meat that is not organic, opt for a vegetarian dish instead, or wild caught fish

- Try to avoid lettuce and berries that are not organic, both are high in pesticides when produced conventionally. Opt for something with a hard skin, such as pineapple if choosing a fruit, and a denser veggie, such as root veggies, which don't require as much pesticides during farming.

It may seem like a lot to remember at first, but just do the best you can, and keep referring back to this list to jog your memory when needed. Eventually, these choices will become second nature and you won't have to put so much effort into remembering what you need to do. And try not to feel overwhelmed, but rather focus on enjoying your dinner and company. Even one small step in the right direction helps; if we try to do everything perfectly, we only create more stress for ourselves, and that's counterproductive to what you're trying to accomplish.

Chapter Six | Toxic Habit # 2: "Relaxing" with Alcohol

I remember when I worked on Wall Street, my favorite thing to do after a long, exhausting, stressful day at work was to unwind with a nice glass of red wine. Of course, I couldn't buy a single glass at the liquor store, so I'd have to buy a bottle. And since I had a bottle, and it was so good, and I could finally relax, I'd usually end up drinking more than just one glass, or two, or three…you get the point.

And by that point, I didn't feel like cooking dinner, I just wanted to relax - I'd worked so hard all day! But I was hungry. So I'd usually grab an Amy's Organic Pizza (frozen) and just pop it in the oven. I got the veggie lovers, so that was ok, right? Getting my veggies in. Oh but then that was so good, and I was so hungry, so I'd end up eating most of it by myself, since I lived alone. But then I really wanted a sweet treat afterward, I'd worked so hard today and put up with so much, I deserved a treat, didn't I?

Besides, if I can't enjoy anything during my day, like my job, I should at least make sure I enjoy what I'm doing at night. So I'd get some vegan coconut based ice cream, that's not so bad, right? So after my organic veggie lover's pizza and wine, I'd sometimes end up eating almost the entire pint of vegan ice cream. And you know, surprisingly, after all that, I don't remember being particularly stuffed. Hmm. What's going on here?

Since I was so strung out from work, the wine would help me to fall asleep; without it I'd be up tossing and turning and staring at the ceiling all night. But even though it helped me to doze off, I never felt well rested when I woke up. In fact, I felt utterly exhausted. And so I'd go through my day, exhausted and miserable, hating what I was doing, and feeling like crap while I was doing it. And the cycle continued.

What's Going On Here?

Let's use my situation as a case study, shall we?

First off, I was using alcohol as a way to decompress after work, which is a recipe for disaster. I was also using it as a way to fall asleep rather than be up half the night from insomnia.

Studies show that while drinking alcohol in the evening can initially help one to fall asleep faster, it ends up disrupting sleep during the second half of the night as it is metabolized and withdrawal symptoms kick in. Some of the ways in which it does this is that it causes less REM sleep (which is thought to be the most mentally restorative), it can lead to more shallow sleep and multiple awakenings, and it can cause more vivid dreams and nightmares, sweating, and overall more stimulation during sleep. This is why people often feel exhausted when they drink before bed, as was my case.

Ayurveda offers many options for managing insomnia, and if I'd been aware of these at the time, perhaps I wouldn't have relied on alcohol to do the trick. I've found that one of the most effective practices for help falling asleep is to develop an nightly meditation routine. Usually, in the case of insomnia, the mind is running wild instead of settling down to fall asleep. By simply focusing on the breath, and concentrating one's awareness, the many thoughts that are racing through the mind may start to reside and sleep will come more easily. It takes practice, but it's worth it.

Another way to help fall asleep faster at night is to develop an evening routine. Here are some of my favorite tips for establishing a routine to help get you to sleep faster and to sleep more soundly:

- About an hour before bed, shut off all screens including computer screens, tablets, phones, etc.

- Lower the lights and create an atmosphere of peace. You can light candles, put on relaxing music, whatever helps you create a calm environment.

- Aromatherapy is very powerful and works on the level of the subconscious mind to help us relax and unwind. Try lavender or a special blend designed for sleep. You can use it in a diffuser, or make your own by filling a bowl with hot water and pouring a few drops of the oil in it.

- Do a full body massage, known as *abhyanga*, with an herbalized oil for sleep (more details are provided later in this chapter). Visit www.TheWisdomOfWellness.com/Resources for recommendations on oils. If you don't have time to do your whole body, at the very least, do the soles of your feet, and optionally your head.

- Have a glass of warm milk about a half hour before bed. Heat it on the stove until it comes to a gentle boil, then turn it off and add a pinch of nutmeg. Allow it to cool to a drinkable temperature and enjoy. There are properties in both the milk and the nutmeg to help encourage peaceful sleep.

- Take a warm bath or shower.

- Try to go to bed at the same time each day to get your body on a regular routine, which will make falling asleep easier.

- Aim to be sleeping as close to 10pm as possible. After 10pm, pitta dosha takes over and we may get a burst of energy or "second wind" that may make it difficult to fall asleep.

- Practice alternate nostril pranayama.

- For additional assistance falling asleep, consider an herbal supplement. Ayurvedic herbs are not addictive and can be used to help us get back on a good sleep schedule. Visit www.TheWisdomOfWellness.com/Resources for recommendations on my favorite night time herbs.

A nightly routine can not only help one fall asleep, but also stay asleep and get better quality sleep. It might seem like it takes a significant time commitment as you first get started, but take a moment to consider what you would be doing instead, and if it's really the best use of your time. Perhaps you enjoy watching television at night. This is not really a productive activity, and the lights from the screen can throw off sleep cycles.

Once you get into the habit of doing these practices, you might really enjoy them, and prefer them over t.v. In addition, once you are sleeping better, you will find that you have more energy and are more efficient during the day, which will actually save you time. So instead of looking at the immediate time commitment required, try to view it from a much broader perspective and see all of the benefits that can result when we prioritize our sleep.

Sleep also affects the nervous system, and without proper sleep, the nervous system becomes strained and this affects our mood and our ability to deal with stress. So in effect, we are making the situation worse by leaving ourselves sleep deprived. Something that may have started out as a small annoyance can over time seem like a big problem, solely based on our body's dampened ability to deal with the situation.

In addition to affecting our ability to sleep soundly, alcohol depresses the central nervous system (made up of the brain and spinal cord), which is what regulates mood and emotions. If we drink to relax instead of observing and processing our emotions, they will still be there when the alcohol wears off. We are not solving the issue, only pushing it aside and burying it deeper into our minds, hearts and physiology.

Another downside to drinking alcohol is that it often lowers one's ability to stick to healthy food choices. In my case, I thought I was being somewhat healthy by eating "organic" frozen pizza, but as we've learned in Chapter 3, frozen food is void of *prana* and many vital nutrients. Also, that coconut ice cream I was eating – full of sugar!! And it is not good for digestion due to the extreme cold nature. By putting both sugar and something very cold into my stomach right after a meal, I was causing all sorts of trouble in my gut.

No wonder I couldn't lose weight! There I was, thinking I was making healthy food choices, and not realizing that the stuff I was eating was very processed, even though it was labeled "organic", it was void of life force and low on nutrients, and it was awful for my digestion. Plus, I was drinking copious amounts of wine, which is also high in sugar and calories, which my body didn't need.

To make matters even worse, I was sitting at a desk all day at work, and not exercising. (Not that exercise is a free pass to eat this way). The lack of movement only added to my digestive weakness, and hence the reason I suffered from constant gas, bloating, and constipation.

So I was walking around in pain all day (from gas), full of toxins, and sleep deprived. If that wouldn't put someone in a bad mood, I don't know what would! No wonder I wanted to drink when I got home. Do you see the vicious cycle that I created for myself??

Now, we can't put the blame on external circumstances, such as our jobs. As we've learned in Chapter 2, we create our own reality. It is within our power to take control of our emotions and thoughts to change our situation. But it requires a certain level of awareness. At the time, I did not have that awareness. I felt as if I were a victim of my environment, as I'm sure many men and women do.

I am so grateful that someone finally spoke up and woke me up! Once I had that inkling of awareness and that I was in control of my life, it led me to take steps to understand what I needed to do in order to change it. And look where that led me – to a career that I absolutely love - helping others to do the same! So if you feel like things are hopeless, please don't give up. It may feel like things are beyond your control, and some unfortunately are, but in many cases we can make a change, which begins by shifting our perspective.

Relaxation and Stress Management

Stress Management is a crucial part of any health regimen, including our efforts to lose weight. The effect of stress on our weight might not be apparent at first, so I'd like to give some context to the process briefly:

When we perceive something as stressful, whether it is actually happening, or we are just thinking about it, the body begins the stress response. I won't get too technical for the purposes of this book, but basically, it involves triggering specific organs in the brain (the thalamus and the hypothalamus) that cause stress hormones to be released (epinephrine and cortisol), and the sympathetic nervous system prepares the body for "fight or flight".

As a result, heart rate increases, more blood is pumped into the muscles, immune function is impaired, as well as the digestive and reproductive systems, as the body is focusing all of its efforts on the impending "fight" or "flight", and therefore ushers energy away from these other systems which are not needed at the moment.

This is fine if it's only a momentary response and our bodies return to a more balanced state shortly thereafter, as that is what this stress response was designed for; however, many of us live in a constant state of moderate to severe stress.

When this is the case, the body's immune, digestive, and reproductive systems are constantly debilitated. When left unchecked, this can eventually lead to weight gain and disease.

It is said that roughly 90% of disease originates from stress. These include ulcers, IBS, diarrhea and constipation, hardening of the arteries, heart attacks, diabetes, PMS, colds and flus, low libido, and more.*

The physiological responses that take place also stimulate areas in the brain that lead us to experience more fear and anger, leading to symptoms of anxiety, depression, and trouble concentrating.

None of this is conducive to weight loss. If you are feeling down with low energy, a poor digestive system, and other complications, you likely won't feel like making healthy food choices or exercising.

There are so many things in life that you feel may be causing you stress – work, family, other responsibilities – so what does one do?

Well, the good news is that our level of stress is a direct result of how we perceive the world. Huh? In other words, we control our reactions to outside stimuli, and thereby determine the level of stress we experience.

So instead of using alcohol to relax, I would like to share some of the amazing techniques I've learned over the years that I find profound transformative. When practiced on a regular basis, these can help us let go of the reliance on alcohol as a means of decompressing. The techniques I will cover include:

- Deep Breathing

- Rotation of Consciousness

- Abhyanga

- Awareness

Deep Breathing

At the beginning of Chapter 1, we did an exercise where we got ourselves into the proper position to allow the breath to deepen and become more full and complete. This is important, because often, when we feel stressed, the breath tends to become more shallow and incomplete. This only perpetuates the situation, because as a result, you are not getting the proper amount of both oxygen and *prana* to allow us to feel good.

You may feel low energy, your digestion can suffer, your mood will suffer, and toxins will build up in the body. This can all contribute to weight gain.

Deep breathing on the other hand, releases tensions, allows oxygen and *prana* to circulate throughout the body, nourishing and enlivening it; it allows your bodily systems to function more efficiently, and can allow your muscles to relax. It is a form of *pranayama*, or control of the vital life force (*prana*) through the breath.

So whenever you begin to feel stressed, I encourage you to take a few moments to sit up tall and take a few deep breaths.

You can also choose to exhale forcefully through your mouth, letting out a sigh as you do so. This can help you to release tensions even further.

Rotation of Consciousness

A great way to help reduce the stress response is to consciously move your awareness throughout your body. You can do this either lying down or sitting up. Start by sending your awareness throughout the different parts of your body, beginning at the top of your head and working your way down to your toes, and as you send your awareness into each part of the body, feel it begin to soften and relax.

Once you've worked your way down, you can then move your awareness back up, starting at your toes, and finishing at the top of your head.

You may want to experiment with working through the front side of your body, and then the back; or doing the left side and then the right.

This practice is an excellent way to begin to focus your mind and clear the thoughts that are causing you to feel stressed. As you relax your body deeper and deeper, the stress will simply start to fall away.

Abhyanga

In Ayurveda, there is a technique known as *Abhyanga*, or self-massage. When performed regularly, it can help to calm and soothe your mind and emotions, bringing with it a sense of grounding and nourishment. This is can often provide the nourishment and satisfaction you are seeking that lead to emotional eating, thereby reducing unhealthy cravings for food.

It's a very intimate practice, getting to know and love your body as you nurture it with warm, healing oils. It helps us to connect your body to your mind and emotions – the disconnection often being a reason for turning to food for comfort.

For this technique, a specific type of oil is chosen based on your unique constitution. Ideally, it should be gently warmed, either using a double boiler method, or by placing a jar of oil in a cup of hot water until it warms.   Then, using a small amount of oil, and starting with the scalp, give yourself a massage, working your way down your body. Make sure to focus a little extra time on any areas that are holding tension, such as the neck and shoulders.

You can use long strokes on the limbs, and a circular motion around the joints. For the stomach, move in the direction of the intestines by starting at the upper right, directly under your rib cage, moving your hands across your stomach to the left, then down, then across to the right.

Visit www.TheWisdomOfWellness.com/Resources for a link to download a PDF of the entire process, as well as recommendations on which oils are best for you.

This is not only very relaxing, but can help improve digestion and elimination if done regularly.

The act of massaging the skin releases "feel good" chemicals such as serotonin. It also improves circulation and facilitates the release of toxins.

It should be performed each morning, about ten minutes before your shower, or in the evening, before a warm bath or shower.

To keep the bathroom drains clear of oil, pour a couple of cups of hot water mixed with a half of cup of vinegar down the drain once a week.

Awareness

Finally, a simple practice that can help you start to better manage your stress response is to bring awareness to the situation. When you feel like you are becoming stressed by something, to mentally take a step back and observe the situation from more of a detached perspective.

Detached doesn't mean that you don't care, but rather, by taking a more objective perspective, even if for only a moment, you will be able to view the situation more clearly, and see things you might have missed before due to the flood of emotions that had been taking over.

By becoming the observer, you can take a more 'holistic' view of the situation, which will in turn allow you to empathize with the other party(s) involved and can ultimately remove the stress you feel now that you can see and understand all of the elements better.

This technique may take some practice, so don't feel discouraged if you're not able to do it right away. Simply try again next time, and each time you may see that you are able to bring your full awareness into the situation sooner than you did the last, and each time, you will be able to more quickly overcome the stress response before it takes hold, leading to a more peaceful, understanding way of being.

Additional Ways to Unwind

In addition to the methods I outlined above, there are plenty of other things you can do to relax and unwind instead of resorting to alcohol:

- Exercise (which can also help break the addiction to alcohol. John Ratey talks about this in *Spark*).

- Meditation

- Talking to or visiting a friend

- Reading an uplifting book

- Watching an inspiring documentary

- Playing with pets (or if you don't have pets, you can volunteer at a local animal shelter)

- Playing with kids

- Playing like a kid!

And the list goes on. Sometimes, when you are feeling down or stressed about your life, it helps to take the focus off of yourself, and instead, look to helping others. Not to push the emotions aside, but to focus on helping those in need rather than allowing yourself to wallow in your sorrows. By shifting the focus to serving, it can become easier to let go of whatever was bringing you down, and allow you to focus on all the blessings you have instead.

To this extent, volunteer work can be very therapeutic. You can go to volunteermatch.org, or another local volunteer organization to find opportunities that might be a good fit for you. When you spend your time serving others, not only does it make a profound impact on their lives, but yours as well.

A Final Note on Alcohol

Alcohol plays a big role in our society – from social gatherings, dinners, trips to the winery, during recreational activities, etc. And it's fine when taken in moderation and with no negative effects.

However, if you feel like alcohol is affecting your sleep or contributing to your weight gain, it's time to a take a look at the benefit vs. the side effects. It might take a period of adjustment, but you can still socialize and enjoy the same activities without consuming alcohol, and after refraining for a while, the desire will likely go away once you note how much better you're feeling as a result.

If it's a challenge to be around alcohol and not drink, perhaps you can take a break from the types of environments where alcohol is the main focus for a while. So instead of heading to the bar with your co-workers, maybe you decide to participate in a team sport instead, or suggest another after-work activity that doesn't revolve around drinking.

There are so many amazing activities can be discovered once you break the habit of ending our days with alcohol. You may find that you have more energy, motivation, and desire to learn new things and enjoy new activities. There's a whole world out there waiting for you beyond the bottle – once I discovered this, I never looked back.

Chapter Seven | Toxic Habit # 3: Not Prioritizing Self-Care

When you don't prioritize self-care, you are doing yourself and everyone around you a disservice. Because when you don't feel good, those around you won't feel good. If you focus all of your time on taking care of others, but never take care of yourself, you are eventually going to burn out. There is only so much energy one can give without replenishing.

The reverse is true as well. If you take the appropriate time and measures to nurture yourself, the good feelings you will have will spread like wildfire! Have you ever been in the presence of someone who is just so radiant and full of life that you can't help but pick up the same type of feeling? That's what I'm talking about! That's what you can be and give to others as well.

The 6 Pillars of Weight Loss

Throughout the course of this book , I've covered many different things you can do to optimize self-care. I'd like to sum it up into what I call *The Six Pillars of Weight Loss*.

- Mindset

- Stress Management/Relaxation

- Proper Rest

- Nutrition

- Digestion & Elimination

- Daily Routine

I touched on most of these, beginning with how mindset allows us to create our own reality and either get results or get in our own way; stress and its effect on our body and our ability to lose weight; the importance of proper rest for optimizing digestion, mood, and managing stress levels; the importance of fresh, organic food, prepared with love; I covered multiple ways to enhance digestion and elimination which are crucial to weight management; and I'd like to talk about daily routine a bit more to demonstrate how you can put it all together.

But before we do that, I'd like to briefly explain the *doshas* a little more, including their role in a routine.

The Doshas

Ayurvedic medicine revolves around the concept of the three *doshas*, which are made up of the five elements. Below is a list of the *doshas* and their corresponding elements:

Vata: Space & Air

Pitta: Fire & Water

Kapha: Water & Earth

These three doshas represent everything in the surrounding environment, including people, food, plants, the seasons, etc. A few qualities associated with each are listed below:

Vata: dry, light, rough, cold, mobile

Pitta: hot, oily, sharp, light, liquid

Kapha: sticky, cool, heavy, slow, soft, dense, liquid, oily

*You may note that the qualites 'liquid' and 'oily' overlap with pitta and kapha -, that is because they both contain some of the water element.

74

Each person has some combination of these three elements that make up their unique constitution, but usually one or two stand out most prominently. The same applies to foods that we eat. For example, something like popcorn would be predominantly vata – it's light, dry, airy, and rough. A chili pepper would be pitta since it's hot, and cheese is an example of a kapha type food since it is heavy, dense, and oily.

These *doshas* also correspond to the seasons, with pitta ruling summer; vata ruling fall and the early part of winter, and kapha ruling over late winter and spring. If you think about the qualities we discussed in relation to the seasons, it makes sense.

They also rule over the time of day, and this what can help us to optimize our routine. You see, in Ayurveda, treatment is with opposites. So in order to bring balance to something, we introduce the opposite quality to it. Below is a list of the doshas and the approximate times of day they rule:

Vata: 2 – 6 AM & PM

Pitta: 10 – 2 AM & PM

Kapha: 6 – 10 AM & PM

I should also mention the main functions for each, to help give this even more context:

Vata: Movement; Communication

Pitta: Digestion; Metabolism

Kapha: Lubrication; Structure; Strength

Using this knowledge, we can plan our days so that we keep each of the *doshas* in balance, and utilize them most wisely. For example, as pitta is the dosha that rules digestion, it is recommended that your largest meal of the day be between 11am – 1pm, right when pitta is highest. This will allow for optimum digestion and metabolism of the food.

During kapha hours is the best time to exercise, because kapha tends to be more slow and heavy, and exercise is the perfect way to offset that. *However, please note, it's not advised to do strenuous activity within a few hours before bed, preferably three hours, so that it doesn't disturb our ability to fall asleep. So exercising during the kapha time of morning (6am – 10am) or in the early part of the evening (around 6pm) is best.*

The vata time of day tends to lend itself to creativity, so this is a good time to schedule business meetings, work on projects, and also to meditate. A nice practice is to meditate at the end of the workday when you're transitioning to being home, as it helps to release the tensions from the workday, leaving your mind fresh for your evening activities.

When we get ourselves into the habit of doing things at the same time each day, not only does it set us up to be more successful by our bodies knowing what to expect, but it also helps us stick to our routine. It's easy to push exercise aside if you just say "I'll do it later", because a lot of the time that later never comes.

Instead, if you know that you exercise every day at 7am, it becomes part of your normal routine, and you just do it, instead of thinking about it and putting it off as you let other things get in the way.

Another tip for success – if there's something you really don't like doing, but you know it needs to get done, schedule it for first thing in your day. So for example, if it's exercise that is a challenge for you to stick with, make plans to do it in the morning rather than after work. It will be more likely to get done, and the sense of accomplishment that results will carry with you for the rest of your day.

Daily Routine

Known as *Dinacharya* in Ayurveda, daily routine is an essential component to a well-balanced lifestyle. It starts from the time you wake up until the time you go to sleep, and can help you optimize your day for optimal functioning of body, mind, and spirit.

By getting yourself on a routine, the body has a better idea of what to expect and when. This helps the body prepare for certain things more effectively, such as digesting food. There are also optimal times of the day to do certain activities, such as eat, sleep and exercise, that will bring about the most benefit. Let's go through an example of a basic daily routine:

- Wake up early; express gratitude for the new day and all the potential that lies in it
- Use the restroom; wash your face and brush your teeth; scrape tongue; oil pulling
- Drink a cup of warm water to flush out toxins and encourage a bowel movement
- Perform *abhyanga*
- Shower
- Perform sun salutations, *pranayama* and meditation
- Breakfast (optional)
- Have lunch between 11 - 2, followed by a short walk
- After work – Can take a brisk walk or do other physical activity
- Dinner
- Shut off screens at least an hour before bed and begin evening routine to prep for bed
- Go to bed early, preferably by 10pm

This is a very basic outline for a daily routine, and is not one-size-fits-all. Some constitutions do better with slightly different wake and sleep times (ie, kaphas should wake up earlier, while vatas should sleep a little more); more or less exercise (kaphas generally require more exercise); some don't require breakfast, etc. But it gives you an idea of how you can structure your days for optimal performance.

In general, it's good to wake fairly early, and be in bed as close to 10pm as possible. The hours between 10pm and 2am are the most restorative for sleep, so by taking advantage of this time and sleeping during as much of it as you can, you give your body the best chance to be well rested.

Practices such as meditation and gratitude are effective all the time, but especially so upon first waking and right before going to sleep. It helps to start your day off right, opening you up to wonderful possibilities, and sets your subconscious mind to create deep trans-formation while you sleep.

Seeing the power of a daily routine, I encourage you to plan out your day for tomorrow. I personally am not someone who likes to live within the confines of a strictly planned out schedule, but I do find this technique very useful for getting things accomplished. And just because you have a plan doesn't mean there isn't room for freedom. When you plan your days like this, it actually allows for more free-dom because you don't have to waste time thinking about what to do next, what to eat, when to find time for exercise, etc.

Having a plan is essential to staying on track with a healthy life-style routine and reaching your goals.

Consistency

The key to reaching your weight loss and overall wellness goals is to be consistent. If you try something for a short period of time and give up, you will not get the results you are looking for. And will power is not the solution, as this is only short lived and does not set you up for lasting results. Therefore, it's important to have other tools available for staying on track. We've discussed many of them throughout this book:

- Knowing your "Why"

- Planning in advance

- Taking things one step at a time and not trying to do every-thing all at once

- Creating a routine that will allow you to build new habits

I'd like to cover a couple of other useful practices as well.

Prioritizing

Another key to being consistent is prioritizing. Earlier in the book, we discussed prioritizing something and scheduling it into your calendar as a helpful practice. But many still do not take their health seriously enough to prioritize it, often until it is too late.

Why should your health and wellness be any less important than say, your work? Work is just temporary and jobs change, but you will have only one body for your entire life. It is wise to give it the care and attention it deserves to keep it in its best condition so that you can live a long, fruitful life, full of energy and abundant health.

What good is it to have a certain title at work, or own certain material items if it comes at the expense of your health and you feel too crappy to enjoy it? Putting our health into perspective like this can allow you to see how important it really is.

Community

Another crucial component in staying consistent is the company you keep. Whatever your goals in life, including reaching and maintaining your ideal weight, it's important to surround yourself with others who have the same values and are working toward similar goals.

The people you choose to spend your time with and associate with have a huge impact on your daily habits, your beliefs, and your mindset. If you are constantly around people who don't care about what they put in their bodies, don't care to prioritize their physical ad mental wellbeing, and don't see the value in a healthy lifestyle, I don't care how disciplined you are, it's eventually going to wear on you!

And, if you're just starting out on your journey, it will make it that much more difficult to stick to your new routine, because there will be constant excuses and reasons to fall off track.

I'm not saying you have to ditch all of your friends, but I'm bringing attention to the fact that people are greatly influenced by the people they are around the most. So if you're serious about stepping up your health and losing that weight for good, it would serve you to surround yourself with those who value their own health, practice healthy habits, and live a clean lifestyle.

It will be a great influence, and if others around you are not constantly doing things that bring about self-sabotage, the pull for you to do them will be less as well.

A good way to get started with a community of like-minded people is to join the Let Go and Lose Weight Facebook Group. There we share tips and inspiration, as well as support each other by sharing in community. It's an excellent resource and available to you as a gift for reading this book.

Nourishment on All Levels

Throughout this book I've strived to emphasize the importance of finding balance on all levels as a way to reach your goals and have long-lasting success with them.

This means that not only is it important to make time to procure, prepare and eat healthy food, make time for physical activity, and other self-care practices including meditation and relaxation, but it's also important to nourish yourself on the levels of the mind and soul.

As a human, it is your nature to be constantly learning and exploring. To that end, it is important that you partake in activities that provide some sort of mental stimulation, whether it be a creative pursuit, or something more scholastic in nature. These activities will not only help you to stay mentally acute, but they also nourish the soul. Every being has a unique gift or talent, and I honestly believe that we are meant to express that in order to be truly balanced and fulfilled in our lives.

If you constantly push the urge aside to focus on other things that you feel 'obligated' to do, and don't make time for what your heart yearns for, you are depriving yourself of your hearts desire, and it will only leave you empty and lacking.

If you've been working at a job you don't really feel passionate about, and don't have any hobbies that truly interest you, it might be time to do some soul-searching to figure out what it is that really sparks your flame.

I often help clients with this by providing Vedic Astrology readings. Thousands of years ago, when Ayurveda was originally practiced, astrology was a crucial component, and all *vaidyas* (Ayurvedic Physicians) were also astrologers. It is now making a reemergence, and I am delighted to be a part of it.

Not only can astrology be used medically to see what you are at risk for healthwise, and where our physiological strengths and weaknesses lie, but it is also a very useful tool for gaining insight into the soul's calling. It can provide guidance as to what type of career will be most satisfying, what hidden talents you might have that lie dormant simply because you are not aware of them, and what blocks might be in the way from you fully expressing all the gifts you have to offer.

Not only can it help bring awareness, which is the first step to making change, but it offers remedies which can help you break through the roadblocks and accelerate your path to success.

I've found the inclusion of astrology in my coaching practice to be profoundly useful when working with clients. It helps them foster a keen sense of self-awareness and self-understanding, which allows them to then see how they fit in the world around them and how everything is interconnected. Also, by discovering or re-acknowledging talents and passions, my clients have gone on to find a level of fulfillment they thought was no longer possible previously.

It is truly amazing to see the transformation when someone takes on an activity or direction in life that is deeply meaningful to them. Sometimes this alone can be what is needed for everything else to fall into place.

You see, when you deny our heart's desire, you are denying your true nature and suppressing your soul from expressing itself. This can lead to symptoms such as emotional eating, mental and emotional imbalances, and even physical disease. This is why it's crucial to not only address the physical aspect when trying to lose weight, but all other aspects of the human experience, to include the emotional, mental, and spiritual. Once you find balance in each of these areas, you will experience wholeness, as the fragmentation that brought you into a state of imbalance will be gone.

Caring What Others Think

A final note before I wrap up this chapter. Too often, I have clients tell me that they didn't do certain things I recommended, even though they knew it would help them, because they were concerned about what people would think.

Now, I wasn't asking them to do anything wild and crazy like run down the street in a clown costume, I was simply asking them to do things like bring their small jar of spice mix with them to the restaurant so they could sprinkle it on their food when it arrived. But to my surprise, I've had many people who say they won't do this because they are afraid what others will think.

To that, I have one response – Who cares!?

If you honestly care about what other people will say if you pull out a jar of spices to sprinkle on their food, then it is definitely time to re-prioritize your values. Why should someone's personal opinion come before your health? If you are fully aware of the benefits that these spices will have on you – better digestion and assimilation, decreased symptoms of indigestion, all leading to more physical comfort and weight loss, why would you let someone's curiosity stop you from enjoying these benefits?

Because honestly, most people who ask you what you are doing are simply curios. And who knows, you might even inspire them to want to learn more and do it for themselves! When you think about it in this sense, by setting a good example, you are potentially improving the lives of others around you. Wouldn't it be nice to know that your good habits have led to others improving their well-being also?

Another complaint I get from women is that sometimes their partners can feel intimidated when they set out on a healthy path, and they might make them feel bad about it. In these cases, I explain to them that change is hard for a lot of people, especially when you share a life together. People get into their comfort zones, and when something pulls them out of it, it can be jolting.

The best thing to do in this type of situation is to sit down and explain to your partner what you are doing, and your reasons why. Hopefully they will understand and will want to support you, but if not, you need to know that it's important that you still do what's best for you. As we discussed at an earlier point in the book, you can't continue to take care of others forever without nourishing yourself. It's just not sustainable.

Perhaps you'll want to mention how you feel your new healthy lifestyle will make you a better mother, wife, employee, etc. and how you will actually end up being able to give more in these roles once you are feeling good yourself. If they still don't understand, I encourage you to give it some time and keep up with your new healthy practices. Often, after some initial resistance, those who are close to you and truly care about you may come around. After the initial fear that change brings, they may become inspired to even try some of these new practices themselves.

Of course, I can't make any promises, because I'm not in your household, but I've seen it happen more often than not, so I encourage you to be strong, prioritize your well-being, and stick with it!

I'll tell you a quick story from personal experience to help give some context. When I first decided to make a career switch and I left my job on Wall Street and sold my condo, a kind aunt and uncle invited me to stay with them while I got situated in a new area. At that time, I had already been living an Ayurvedic lifestyle, so that meant cooking my food at home, from scratch, every day.

Let me tell you, they were so surprised by this, because it was so out of the ordinary to them! Their normal meals consisted of something that was either delivered to their doorstep, procured at a restaurant, or pulled out of the freezer and microwaved. The smells of the delicious food and the love and prep that went into making it were completely foreign to them.

At first, they used to tease me about it. I knew it was only due to their ignorance and insecurities, so I didn't find it bothersome, I simply let them tease. Then they wanted to try it. Then they started experimenting with making a couple things here and there. After I moved out of that house, we gathered for a holiday gathering a few years later, and to my utter astonishment, the aunt I had lived with had made not only one, but two healthy, delicious dishes from scratch that she shared at the party!

I was amazed! I was so proud of her, and so delighted that my healthy habits had rubbed off, because now they were taking steps toward improving their own health.

Conclusion

I've hope I was able to provide you with some inspiration from the stories I've shared, and hope you've gained lots of practical advice that you can put into practice immediately to get you closer to your goals.

Most of all, I hope I've been able to show you a new way to approaching weight loss. Gone are the days of struggling with dieting, excessive exercise, and other gimmicks that don't produce long-term results.

Instead, I hope you can see how weight loss is the natural by-product of a balanced, fulfilled life. And through the tools and techniques discussed throughout this book, I hope you have a better idea of what it takes to achieve this balance.

I encourage you to choose just one or two practices that you can implement immediately to get you on your way. And as you progress, you can add an additional practice every week or two. By taking this approach, you can set yourself up for success by making changes gradually. As each one becomes a new habit, you can add more and let go of old habits and beliefs.

If you'd like to receive some additional tips for effortlessly managing your weight, you can get a free copy of my e-book 10 Ways to Lose 10 lbs with Ease by visiting http://bit.ly/1PLQ0DF.

You can also visit my website at www.TheWisdomOfWellness.com where I regularly publish fun and informative articles, which are great for getting new ideas and ongoing motivation. Be sure to visit the "Resources" page for additional free gifts, as well as recommendations for supportive herbal supplements and oils.

Finally, I urge you to do your best, be consistent, and seek support if you need it - you don't have to do it alone. In community you can find support and encouragement toward your goals, as well meet potential life-long friends. Now what could be better than that!

Glossary

Chakras – The energy centers in the body, related to nerve plexus centers, which govern bodily functions. Each chakra is a reservoir of consciousness.

Dosha – The three main psycho-physiological functional principles of the body (vata, pitta, and kapha). They determine each individual's constitution and maintain the integrity of the human body. The *doshas* govern the individual's response to changes. When disturbed, they can initiate the disease process.

Kapha – One of the three doshas, combining the water and earth elements. Kapha is the energy that forms the body's structure – bones, muscles, tendons – and provides the "glue" that holds the cells together. It supplies the water for all bodily parts and systems, lubricates joints, moisturizes the skin, and maintains immunity. In balance, kapha is expressed as love, calmness, and forgiveness. Out of balance, it leads to attachment, greed, and envy.

Pitta – One of the three doshas; it corresponds to the elements of fire and water. Sometimes referred to as the fire or bile principle, pitta governs digestion, absorption, assimilation, metabolism, and body temperature. In balance, pitta promotes understanding and intelligence; out of balance pitta arouses anger, hatred, and jealousy.

Prana – The vital life energy. Without it, life cannot exist. The flow of cellular intelligence from one cell to another. Equivalent to the Oriental *Ch'i* or *Ki*.

Pranayama – The control of life energy by various techniques which regulate and restrain breath, through which one can control the mind and improve one's quality of awareness and perception. Helpful with all types of meditation.

Vata – One of the three doshas, combining the space and air elements; it is the subtle energy associated with bodily movement and governs breathing, blinking, muscle and tissue movement, pulsation of the heart, and all movements in the cytoplasm and cell membranes. In balance, vata promotes creativity and flexibility; out of balance, vata produces fear and anxiety.

Definitions taken from The Complete Book of Ayurvedic Home Remedies, by Vasant Lad, B.A.M.S., M.A.Sc.

www.ingramcontent.com/pod-product-compliance
Lightning Source LLC
Chambersburg PA
CBHW030409290526
45785CB00004B/1946